Free (or Almost Free) Prescription Medications

Where and How to Get Them

Presented and Prepared
by
David Johnson

Robert D. Reed Publishers • San Francisco, CA

Robert D. Reed Publishers
750 La Playa, Suite 647
San Francisco, CA 94121
Phone: 650-994-6570 • Fax: -6579
E-mail: 4bobreed@msn.com
web site: www.rdrpublishers.com

Typesetter: **Barbara Kruger**
Cover Designer: **Julia Gaskill**

ISBN 1-931741-15-8

Library of Congress Catalog Card Number   2002106089

Manufactured, typeset and printed in the United States of America

Low and No Cost Assistance Programs For Prescription Medication

168 assistance programs covering 1,415 prescription medications

Easy to use   Easy to read   Easy to follow

This is the only book offering this information on one of America's best-kept medical secrets.

All programs require: You have no insurance that provides prescription coverage and are ineligible for State Medicaid programs.

They all have income guidelines but only 13 require your income to be less than $715.00 per month (based on a single person household).

Most of the programs allow incomes between $1,070.00 and $3,210.00 per month (based on a single-person household).

This book is filled with potential livesaving information.

I would like to take a moment and give a special thank you to the people who helped this project truly come to life:

Grandma and Gwenn for their divine guidance and intervention.

Dr. Richard Craft, Sr., M.D., and his staff for helping to prove these programs do work.

Dr. Jose Padin, PhD., for convincing me to take the necessary last step in bringing this project to life.

A special thank you to Cheryl, for keeping the fires of faith and hope burning when I couldn't, and for not letting me surrender to my own foolish beliefs. If not for this, this project would still be hidden on a computer disk.

To all of us in the same leaky boat...

Low and No Cost Assistance Programs For Prescription Medication has taken over 2-1/2 years of research to complete. This 230-page book contains information on 168 assistance programs involving 1,415 prescriptions medications obtainable at little or no cost to qualifying individuals. All of the programs require that you have no insurance providing prescription coverage and are ineligible for State Medicaid programs. They all have income guidelines, but only 13 require your income to be less than $715.00 per month (based on a single-person household). Most of the programs allow incomes between $1,070.00 and $3,210.00 per month (based on a single-person household).

This started as a project of self-desperation. I have MS. In 1999, I lost my insurance coverage. At that time, my monthly drug bill was in excess of $1,500.00 per month, which exceeded my monthly fixed income. So, I went looking for alternatives. I went to all of the usual places: county, state, federal, and private social services agencies, my doctors, and anyone else I could think of, that may have had an answer. No one had a reasonable answer, except: *"You've found one of the many cracks in our healthcare system."*

In a last desperate attempt, I contacted one of the drug manufacturers and to my surprise; they had an assistance program. I figured if one manufacturer had a program, others might have a program as well. Through these programs, I was able to reduce my monthly drug bill to a reasonable $100.00 per month.

In the hunt for funding, I was told: *"There is no funding available for a project of this nature."* *"We will consider some funding but we will have to have the final say on the contents, presentation of the material and it will have to be published under our name."* I am proud of the fact this project has been completed through the efforts of volunteers and financed by using their own money.

The other theme heard: *"The committee has determined the project has no value."* *"We question the need for a project like this."* A few others and I have always believed in the need and value of this project, because no one should have to decide between health and a place to live or food to eat. As I was told, *"We can't help with your health care but we do have programs to help if you do become homeless."*

This is a guide sort of like a road map. We have tried to provide as much information as possible to allow you to contact the various program providers. If you do not find your medication, contact your local pharmacy to find out the manufacturer of that medication.

Then give the manufacturer a call. They MAY or MAY NOT have a program.

No matter how good or complete you think you have done something, someone always has an idea after all is thought to be complete. Those of you working with this manual will encounter changes in these programs faster than I will encounter the changes. If you find the programs have changed, would you please e-mail this information to me at KMAFoundation@excite.com, it would be greatly appreciated. If you know of a program that has not been included in this edition forward it and I will put it in the next edition.

Most of these programs do take a certain amount of time to get started. Do not get discouraged. I hope you find this information useful, beneficial, and helpful in improving your ability to have a better quality of life.

Sincerely,

David Johnson

2001 FEDERAL POVERTY GUIDELINES FOR THE 48 CONTIGUOUS STATES AND THE DISTRICT OF COLUMBIA

Number In Family	Gross Yearly Income*	Gross Monthly Income	Approximate Hourly Wage**
1	$8,590.00	$714.46	$4.13
2	$11,616.00	$966.14	$5.58
3	$14,630.00	$1,216.82	$7.03
4	$17,650.00	$1,468.00	$8.49
5	$20,670.00	$1,719.19	$9.94
6	$23,690.00	$1,970.37	$11.39
7	$26,710.00	$2,221.55	$12.84
8	$29,730.00	$2,472.74	$14.29
Over 8 add for Each child	$3,020.00	$251.18	$1.45

150% of 2001 FEDERAL POVERTY GUIDELINES FOR THE 48 CONTIGUOUS STATES AND THE DISTRICT OF COLUMBIA

Number In Family	Gross Yearly Income*	Gross Monthly Income	Approximate Hourly Wage**
1	$12,885.00	$1,071.69	$6.19
2	$17,424.00	$1,449.21	$8.38
3	$21,945.00	$1,825.23	$10.55
4	$26,475.00	$2,202.01	$12.73
5	$31,005.00	$2,578.78	$14.91
6	$35,535.00	$2,955.56	$17.08
7	$40,065.00	$3,332.33	$19.26
8	$44,595.00	$3,709.10	$21.44
Over 8 add for Each child	$4,530.00	$376.77	$2.18

200% of 2001 FEDERAL POVERTY GUIDELINES FOR THE 48 CONTIGUOUS STATES AND THE DISTRICT OF COLUMBIA

Number In Family	Gross Yearly Income*	Gross Monthly Income	Approximate Hourly Wage**
1	$17,180.00	$1,428.91	$8.26
2	$23,232.00	$1,932.28	$11.17
3	$29,260.00	$2,433.64	$14.07
4	$35,300.00	$2,936.01	$16.97
5	$41,340.00	$3,438.38	$19.88
6	$47,380.00	$3,940.74	$22.78
7	$53,420.00	$4,443.11	$25.68
8	$59,460.00	$4,945.47	$28.59
Over 8 add for Each child	$6,040.00	$502.37	$2.90

250% of 2001 FEDERAL POVERTY GUIDELINES FOR THE 48 CONTIGUOUS STATES AND THE DISTRICT OF COLUMBIA

Number In Family	Gross Yearly Income*	Gross Monthly Income	Approximate Hourly Wage**
1	$21,475.00	$1,786.14	$10.32
2	$29,040.00	$2,415.35	$13.96
3	$36,575.00	$3,042.06	$17.58
4	$44,125.00	$3,670.01	$21.21
5	$51,675.00	$4,297.97	$24.84
6	$59,225.00	$4,925.93	$28.47
7	$66,775.00	$5,553.88	$32.10
8	$74,325.00	$6,181.84	$35.73
Over 8 add for Each child	$7,550.00	$627.96	$3.63

Source: *Federal Register v.665 n.3, 2/15, 2001 pp.7555-7557*
*Rounded off to nearest dollar amount
**Based on full-time employment of 2080 hours per year

ALPHABETICAL LISTING

OF

PROGRAM PROVIDERS

ALPHABETICAL LISTING

OF

PHARMACEUTICAL COMPANIES WITHOUT PROGRAMS

We have included these companies even though, at this time, they do not have an assistance program. They have had programs in the past, however. If your medication is manufactured by one of these companies, give them a call or write them a letter. They may offer some assistance.

Alpha Therapeutics
5555 Valley Blvd.
Los Angeles, CA 90033
1-800-421-0008

Alpharma
7205 Windsor Blvd.
Baltimore, MD 21244
1-800-638-9096

Alra Laboratories
3850 Clearview Court
Gurnee, IL 60031
1-800-248-2572

Barre-National, Inc.
7205 Windsor Rd.
Baltimore, MD 21244
1-410-298-1000

Bedford Laboratories
300 Northfield Rd.
Bradford, OH 44146
1-887-324-4248

Braintree Laboratories
P.O. Box 850929
Braintree, MA 02185
1-781-843-2202

Dailahi Pharmaceuticals
11 Philips Parkway
Montvale, NJ 07645
1-887-324-4246

Dey Laboratories
2750 Napa Valley Corp Drive
Napa, CA 94558
1-800-755-5560

Dura-Med Pharmaceuticals
5040 Dura Med Drive
Cincinnati, OH 45213
1-800-543-8338

Endo Laboratories
233 Willington West Chester Pike
Chads Ford, PA 19317
1-80-462-3636

Faro Pharmaceuticals, Inc.
135 Route 202/206
Bedminster, NJ 07921
1-877-994-3276

Ion Laboratories
743 Pebble Drive
Fort Worth, TX 76118
1-817-284-8044

Lotus Biochemical
P.O. Box 3586
Radford, VA. 24143
1-800-455-5525

Lunsco
Route 2, Box 62
Pulaski, VA 24301
1-540-980-4358

Merz Pharmaceutical
4215 Tudor Lane
Greensboro, NC 27410
1-910-856-2000

Mission Pharmaceutical Company
10999-1H 10 West
Suite 1000
San Antonio, TX 78730
1-800-292-7364

Mylan Pharmaceuticals
781 Chestnut Ridge Rd.
P.O. Box 4310
Morgantown, WV 26504
1-800-635-5067

Novopharm USA, Inc.
165 E Commerce Dr. 100-201
Schaumberg, IL 60173
1-800-635-5067

Ohmeda Pharmaceuticals
110 Allen Rd.
Liberty Corner, NJ 07938
1-800-345-2708

Polymedica
11 State St.
Woburn MA 01801
1-800-536-8745

Savage Laboratories
60 Baylis Rd
Melville, NY 11747
1-800-231-0206 ext. 3047

Schwarz Parma, Inc.
5600 W. Country Lane Rd.
P.O. Box 2038
Milwaukee, WI 53201
1-800-558-5115

Teva Pharmaceuticals
650 Cathill Rd.
Sellsville, PA 18960
1-800-838-2872

Watson Labs.
311 Bonnie Circle
Corona, CA 91720
1-800-272-5525

Warner Chilcott Laboratories, Inc.
Rockaway 80 Corporate Circle
100 Enterprise Dr.
Rockaway, NJ 07986
1-800-521-8813

ALPHABETICAL LISTING

OF

MEDICATIONS

MEDICATION	Page	PROGRAM PROVIDER
8-MOP Capsules	144	ICN Pharmaceuticals, Inc.
Abelcet	158	Liposome Company, Inc.
Accolate	79	AstraZeneca Foundation
Accupril	187	Warner-Lambert
Accuretic	199	Roche Laboratories
Accuretic	187	Warner-Lambert
Accutane	199	Roche Laboratories
Acebutolol HCL	223	Wyeth-Ayerst Laboratories
ACI-Jel	180	Ortho-McNeil Pharm.
Aclovate Cream	137	Glaxo Wellcome, Inc.
Aclovate Lotion	137	Glaxo Wellcome, Inc.
Acthar Gel	172	NORD
Acthrel	126	Ferring Pharmaceuticals, Inc.
Actigall	134	Geneva Pharmaceuticals
Actimmune	149	InterMune Pharmaceuticals
Activase	132	Genentech, Inc.
Actos	215	Takeda Pharmaceuticals
Adalat	89	Bayer Pharmaceutical
Adalat CC	89	Bayer Pharmaceutical
ADEKs Pediatric Drops	84	Axcan-Scandipharm, Inc.
Adenoscan	128	Fujisawa USA, Inc.
Adriamycin	192	Pharmacia & Upjohn
Adrucil	192	Pharmacia & Upjohn
Aerobid Inhaler System	127	Forest Pharmaceuticals, Inc.
Aerobid-M Inhaler System	127	Forest Pharmaceuticals, Inc.
AeroChamber	127	Forest Pharmaceuticals, Inc.
AeroChamber with Mask	127	Forest Pharmaceuticals, Inc.
Agenerase Capsules	137	Glaxo Wellcome, Inc.
Agenerase Oral	137	Glaxo Wellcome, Inc.
Aggrastat Injectable	165	Merck & Company
Aggrastat Premix Injectable	165	Merck & Company
Aggrenox	97	Boehringer Ingelheim
Agrylin	198	Roberts Pharmaceutical
Agrylin	211	Shire Pharmaceuticals
Albuterol Sulfate	223	Wyeth-Ayerst Laboratories
Aldactazide	209	Searle & Co.
Aldactone	209	Searle & Co.

MEDICATION	Page	PROGRAM PROVIDER
Anaprox Tabs	199	Roche Laboratories
Ancobon	144	ICN Pharmaceuticals, Inc.
Antabuse	223	Wyeth-Ayerst Laboratories
Antivert	189	Pfizer Pharmaceutical, Inc.
Antivert 25 mg Tabs	189	Pfizer Pharmaceutical, Inc.
Antivert 50 mg Tabs	189	Pfizer Pharmaceutical, Inc.
Anturane	134	Geneva Pharmaceuticals
Anusol-HC 2.5% Crème	168	Monarch Pharmaceuticals
Anusol-HC Suppositories	168	Monarch Pharmaceuticals
Anzemet	83	Aventis-Oncology Pact Prg.
Anzemet	141	Hoechst Marion Roussel
Apresazide	134	Geneva Pharmaceuticals
Apresoline	134	Geneva Pharmaceuticals
Aralen	203	Sanofi Pharmaceuticals, Inc.
Arava	139	Hoechst Marion Roussel,Inc.
Aredia	134	Geneva Pharmaceuticals
Aredia	174	Novartis Pharmaceuticals
Aricept	190	Pfizer Pharmaceuticals
Arimidex	79	AstraZeneca Foundation
Aristocort Cream A .01%	128	Fujisawa USA, Inc.
Aristocort Cream A .025%	128	Fujisawa USA, Inc.
Aristocort Cream A .5%	128	Fujisawa USA, Inc.
Aristocort Ointment A .1%	128	Fujisawa USA, Inc.
Aristocort Suspension	128	Fujisawa USA, Inc.
Armour Thyroid	127	Forest Pharmaceuticals, Inc.
Aromasin	192	Pharmacia & Upjohn
Artane	223	Wyeth-Ayerst Laboratories
Artane Elixir	156	Lederle Labs
Artane Tabs	156	Lederle Labs
Arthrotec	209	Searle & Co.
Asacol	194	Proctor & Gamble Pharm.
Asenden	156	Lederle Labs
Atacand	76	AstraZeneca LP, Inc.
Atarax Syrup	189	Pfizer Pharmaceutical, Inc.
Atarax Tabs	189	Pfizer Pharmaceutical, Inc.
Atenolol	74	Apothecon-Bristol-Myers
Atromid S	223	Wyeth-Ayerst Laboratories

MEDICATION	Page	PROGRAM PROVIDER
Atropine Sulfate	119	Eli Lilly and Company
Atrovent Inhalation Aerosol	97	Boehringer Ingelheim
Atrovent Inhalation Solution	97	Boehringer Ingelheim
Atrovent Nasal Spray 0.03%	97	Boehringer Ingelheim
Atrovent Nasal Spray 0.06%	97	Boehringer Ingelheim
Augmentin Chewable Tabs	212	SmithKline Beecham, Inc.
Augmentin Oral Concentrate	212	SmithKline Beecham, Inc.
Auralgan Optic Solution	223	Wyeth-Ayerst Laboratories
Avalide	100	Bristol-Myers Foundation
Avandia	212	SmithKline Beecham, Inc.
Avapro	100	Bristol-Myers Foundation
Aventyl HCL Liquid	119	Eli Lilly and Company
Aventyl HCL Pulvules	119	Eli Lilly and Company
Avonex	95	Biogen
Axid	119	Eli Lilly and Company
Aygestin	123	ESI Lederle, Inc.
Aygestin	223	Wyeth-Ayerst Laboratories
Azmacort Inhaler Aerosol	196	Rhone Poulenc Rorer, Inc.
Azopt Oral Suspension	64	Alcon Labs
Baclofen	137	Glaxo Wellcome, Inc.
Bactrim Tabs	199	Roche Laboratories
Bactrim DS Tabs	199	Roche Laboratories
Bactrim Pediatric Suspension	199	Roche Laboratories
Bactroban Cream	212	SmithKline Beecham, Inc.
Bactroban Nasal	212	SmithKline Beecham, Inc.
Beclovent Inhalation Aerosol	137	Glaxo Wellcome, Inc.
Beconase AQ Nasal Spray	137	Glaxo Wellcome, Inc.
Beconase Inhalation System	137	Glaxo Wellcome, Inc.
Beelith	91	Beach Pharmaceuticals
Benoquin Cream	144	ICN Pharmaceuticals, Inc.
Bentyl Capsules	139	Hoechst Marion Roussel,Inc.
Bentyl Syrup	139	Hoechst Marion Roussel,Inc.
Bentyl Tabs	139	Hoechst Marion Roussel,Inc.
Benzagel 5 Acne Gel	112	Dermik Laboratories
Benzagel 10 Acne Gel	112	Dermik Laboratories
Benzamycin Gel	112	Dermik Laboratories
Benzashave Cream	161	Medicis Pharmaceutical

MEDICATION	Page	PROGRAM PROVIDER
Capital Oral Suspension	70	Amarin Pharmaceuticals
Capitrol Shampoo	221	Westwood-Squibb Pharm.
Capoten	100	Bristol-Myers Foundation
Capoten	185	Par Pharmaceuticals, Inc.
Capozide	100	Bristol-Myers Foundation
Carafate Suspension	139	Hoechst Marion Roussel,Inc.
Carafate Syrup	139	Hoechst Marion Roussel,Inc.
Carafate Tabs	139	Hoechst Marion Roussel,Inc.
Cardene	199	Roche Laboratories
Cardene SR	199	Roche Laboratories
Cardizem	139	Hoechst Marion Roussel,Inc.
Cardizem CD	139	Hoechst Marion Roussel,Inc.
Cardizem SR	139	Hoechst Marion Roussel,Inc.
Cardura	189	Pfizer Pharmaceutical, Inc.
Carnitor	172	NORD
Casodex	79	AstraZeneca Foundation
Cataflam	134	Geneva Pharmaceuticals
Catapres-TTS patches ONLY	97	Boehringer Ingelheim
Caverject	192	Pharmacia & Upjohn
Ceclor Pulvules	119	Eli Lilly and Company
Ceclor Suspension	119	Eli Lilly and Company
CeeNU	99	Bristol-Myers Access
Cefaclor	223	Wyeth-Ayerst Laboratories
Cefizox	128	Fujisawa USA, Inc.
Ceftin	137	Glaxo Wellcome, Inc.
Cefzil Oral Suspension	100	Bristol-Myers Foundation
Cefzil Tabs	100	Bristol-Myers Foundation
Celebrex 100 mg	209	Searle & Co.
Celebrex 200 mg	209	Searle & Co.
Celestone	205	Schering Labs/Key Pharm.
Celexa	127	Forest Pharmaceuticals, Inc.
CellCept Capsules	199	Roche Laboratories
CellCept Oral Suspension	199	Roche Laboratories
CellCept Tabs	199	Roche Laboratories
Celluvisc Lubricant Eye Drops	65	Allergan Pharmaceuticals,Inc.
Cephalexin	74	Apothecon-Bristol-Myers
Cephalexin Oral Suspension	74	Apothecon-Bristol-Myers

MEDICATION	Page	PROGRAM PROVIDER
Cephulac 10 gm	139	Hoechst Marion Roussel,Inc.
Cephulac 15 ml	139	Hoechst Marion Roussel,Inc.
Ceptaz	137	Glaxo Wellcome, Inc.
Cerebyx	187	Warner-Lambert
Cerezyme	135	Genzyme Therapeutics
Cetacaine Topical	109	Cetylite Industries, Inc.
Chibroxin	163	Merck & Company
Chlo-Amine	89	Bayer Pharmaceutical
Chronulac Lactulose Syrup	139	Hoechst Marion Roussel,Inc.
Cilest	150	Janssen Pharmaceutica
Cimetidine	223	Wyeth-Ayerst Laboratories
Cinobac	178	Oclassen Dermatologics,Inc.
Cipro	89	Bayer Pharmaceutical
Cipro IV	89	Bayer Pharmaceutical
Cipro Oral Suspension	89	Bayer Pharmaceutical
Citrolith	91	Beach Pharmaceuticals
Claforan	139	Hoechst Marion Roussel,Inc.
Claritin D-12 Retabs	205	Schering Labs/Key Pharm.
Claritin Retabs	205	Schering Labs/Key Pharm.
Claritin Syrup	205	Schering Labs/Key Pharm.
ClaritinTabs	205	Schering Labs/Key Pharm.
Climara	92	Berlex Laboratories
Clindamycin Injectable	76	AstraZeneca LP, Inc.
Clinoril	163	Merck & Company
Clomid	139	Hoechst Marion Roussel,Inc.
Clonidine HCL	223	Wyeth-Ayerst Laboratories
Clorpes	94	Bertek Pharmaceuticals,Inc.
Clozaril	174	Novartis Pharmaceuticals
Clozaril	176	Novartis (Sandoz) Pharm.
Codeine Oral Suspension	70	Amarin Pharmaceuticals
Cogard	100	Bristol-Myers Foundation
Cogentin Injectable	163	Merck & Company
Cogentin Tabs	163	Merck & Company
Cognex	143	Horizon Pharmaceuticals
Combivent Inhalation Aerosol	97	Boehringer Ingelheim
Combivir	137	Glaxo Wellcome, Inc.
Compazine Spansules	212	SmithKline Beecham, Inc.

MEDICATION	Page	PROGRAM PROVIDER
Ditropan Tabs	67	Alza Pharmaceuticals
Ditropan XL	67	Alza Pharmaceuticals
Diucardin	223	Wyeth-Ayerst Laboratories
Diuril Capsules	163	Merck & Company
Diuril Oral Suspension	163	Merck & Company
Diuril Tabs	163	Merck & Company
Dobutamine Injectable	76	AstraZeneca LP, Inc.
Dobutrex Solution	119	Eli Lilly and Company
Dolobid	163	Merck & Company
Domepaste Bandages	89	Bayer Pharmaceutical
Donnatal	223	Wyeth-Ayerst Laboratories
Donnazyme	56	A.H. Robins Co.
Dostinex	192	Pharmacia & Upjohn
Dovonex Cream	222	Westwood-Squibb Pharm.
Dovonex Lotion	222	Westwood-Squibb Pharm.
Dovonex Scalp Solution	222	Westwood-Squibb Pharm.
Doxil Injectable	67	Alza Pharmaceuticals
Doxorubicin Injectable	76	AstraZeneca LP, Inc.
Drisdol	203	Sanofi Pharmaceuticals,Inc.
Drithocreme .10% HP Cream	112	Dermik Laboratories
Drithocreme .25% HP Cream	112	Dermik Laboratories
Drithocreme .50% HP Cream	112	Dermik Laboratories
Drithocreme 1.0% HP Cream	112	Dermik Laboratories
Dritho-scalp	112	Dermik Laboratories
Droperidol Injectable	76	AstraZeneca LP, Inc.
DTIC Dome	89	Bayer Pharmaceutical
Duricef	100	Bristol-Myers Foundation
Duragesic Transdermal	150	Janssen Pharmaceutica
Dyazide	212	SmithKline Beecham, Inc.
Dynacin Capsules	161	Medicis Pharmaceutical
Dynacire	121	Eli Lilly and Company
Dynapen	100	Bristol-Myers Foundation
EC Naprosyn Tabs	199	Roche Laboratories
Edecrin	163	Merck & Company
Effexor Tabs	223	Wyeth-Ayerst Laboratories
Effexor XR	223	Wyeth-Ayerst Laboratories
Efudex Cream	144	ICN Pharmaceuticals, Inc.

MEDICATION	Page	PROGRAM PROVIDER
Flovent 220 mcg Inhalation Aerosol	137	Glaxo Wellcome, Inc.
Flovent Nasal Spray	137	Glaxo Wellcome, Inc.
Flovent Rotadisk 50 mcg	137	Glaxo Wellcome, Inc.
Flovent Rotadisk 100 mcg	137	Glaxo Wellcome, Inc.
Flovent Rotadisk 250 mcg	137	Glaxo Wellcome, Inc.
Floxin	180	Ortho-McNeil Pharm.
Fludara	93	Berlex Laboratories
Fluorouracil	199	Roche Laboratories
Fortaz	137	Glaxo Wellcome, Inc.
Fortovase	199	Roche Laboratories
Fosamax	163	Merck & Company
Foscavir	77	AstraZeneca-Foscavir
Fototar Cream	144	ICN Pharmaceuticals, Inc.
Fragmin	192	Pharmacia & Upjohn
FUDR	199	Roche Laboratories
Fulvicin	205	Schering Labs/Key Pharm.
Fungizone	74	Apothecon-Bristol-Myers
Fungizone	99	Bristol-Myers Access
Gabitril	57	Abbott Laboratories
Galzin	131	Gates Pharmaceutical
Gantanol	199	Roche Laboratories
Garamycin Cream	205	Schering Labs/Key Pharm.
Garamycin Gel	205	Schering Labs/Key Pharm.
Garamycin Ophthalmic Solution	205	Schering Labs/Key Pharm.
Gastrocrom Oral Concentrate	160	Medeva Pharmaceuticals,Inc.
Gemzar	119	Eli Lilly and Company
Glacon	64	Alcon Labs
Gliadel Wafers	83	Aventis-Oncology Pact Prg.
Gliadel Wafers	197	Rhone Poulenc Rorer, Inc.
Glucagon	119	Eli Lilly and Company
Glucophage	100	Bristol-Myers Foundation
Glucotrol	189	Pfizer Pharmaceutical, Inc.
Glucotrol XL	189	Pfizer Pharmaceutical, Inc.
Glyset	192	Pharmacia & Upjohn
Grifulvin V Tabs	180	Ortho-McNeil Pharm.
Grisactin Capsules	223	Wyeth-Ayerst Laboratories
Grisactin Tabs	223	Wyeth-Ayerst Laboratories

MEDICATION	Page	PROGRAM PROVIDER
Gyno-Daktarin	150	Janssen Pharmaceutica
Habitrol	134	Geneva Pharmaceuticals
Haldol	150	Janssen Pharmaceutica
Haldol	180	Ortho-McNeil Pharm.
Haldol Deconoate Inject 100mg/ml	180	Ortho-McNeil Pharm.
Haldol Deconoate Inject 50mg/ml	180	Ortho-McNeil Pharm.
Halog Cream	221	Westwood-Squibb Pharm.
Halog Ointment	221	Westwood-Squibb Pharm.
Halog Solution	221	Westwood-Squibb Pharm.
Halotestin	192	Pharmacia & Upjohn
Hemofil-M	88	Baxter Laboratories
Herceptin	132	Genentech, Inc.
Hexalen	220	U.S. Bioscience, Inc.
Hiprex	139	Hoechst Marion Roussel,Inc.
HIVID	199	Roche Laboratories
Humalog	119	Eli Lilly and Company
Humatrope	119	Eli Lilly and Company
Humorsol	163	Merck & Company
Humulin (all types)	119	Eli Lilly and Company
Hydrea	99	Bristol-Myers Access
Hydrocet	70	Amarin Pharmaceuticals
Hydrocet	103	Carnrick Laboratories
Hydrocortone Tabs	163	Merck & Company
HydroDIURIL	163	Merck & Company
Hygroton	196	Rhone Poulenc Rorer, Inc.
Hylorel	160	Medeva Pharmaceuticals,Inc.
Hytakerol	203	Sanofi Pharmaceuticals,Inc.
Hytone Cream	112	Dermik Laboratories
Hytone Lotion	112	Dermik Laboratories
Hytone Ointment	112	Dermik Laboratories
Hyzaar	163	Merck & Company
Idamycin	192	Pharmacia & Upjohn
Iflex/Mesna	99	Bristol-Myers Access
Iletin II Lente	119	Eli Lilly and Company
Iletin II NPH	119	Eli Lilly and Company
Ilosone	113	Dista Products
Ilosone	119	Eli Lilly and Company

MEDICATION	Page	PROGRAM PROVIDER
Isopto Cetapred	64	Alcon Labs
Isopto Homatropine	64	Alcon Labs
Isopto Hyoscine	64	Alcon Labs
Isordil Sublingual Tabs	223	Wyeth-Ayerst Laboratories
Isordil Tembids	223	Wyeth-Ayerst Laboratories
Isordil Titradose	223	Wyeth-Ayerst Laboratories
ITB	172	NORD
Kadian C-11	124	Faulding Laboratories
Kantrex	100	Bristol-Myers Foundation
Kay Ciel Oral Suspension	127	Forest Pharmaceuticals,Inc.
Kay Ciel Powder Packets	127	Forest Pharmaceuticals,Inc.
K-Dur	154	Key Pharmaceuticals
K-Dur	205	Schering Labs/Key Pharm.
Keflex	119	Eli Lilly and Company
Keflex Oral Suspension	113	Dista Products
Keflex Pulvules	113	Dista Products
Keftab	113	Dista Products
Keftab	119	Eli Lilly and Company
Kefurox	119	Eli Lilly and Company
Kemadrin	168	Monarch Pharmaceuticals
Kenalog Capsules	100	Bristol-Myers Foundation
Kenalog Tabs	100	Bristol-Myers Foundation
Kenalog Aerosol Spray	100	Bristol-Myers Foundation
Kenalog Cream	100	Bristol-Myers Foundation
Kenalog Lotion	100	Bristol-Myers Foundation
Kenalog Ointment	100	Bristol-Myers Foundation
Kenalog Pediatric Injection	100	Bristol-Myers Foundation
Kenalog-10	100	Bristol-Myers Foundation
Kenalog-40	100	Bristol-Myers Foundation
Kenalog-in-Orabase	100	Bristol-Myers Foundation
Keppra	217	UCB Pharmaceuticals, Inc.
Kerlone	209	Searle & Co.
Klaron Lotion	112	Dermik Laboratories
Klonopin	199	Roche Laboratories
Klor-Con	219	Upsher-Smith
Klotrix	100	Bristol-Myers Foundation
K-Lyte CL	100	Bristol-Myers Foundation

MEDICATION	Page	PROGRAM PROVIDER
Lipitor	187	Warner-Lambert
Lithobid	214	Solvay Pharmaceuticals,Inc.
Livostin	150	Janssen Pharmaceutica
Locoid Cream	125	Ferndale Laboratories, Inc.
Locoid Lipocream C Cream	125	Ferndale Laboratories, Inc.
Locoid Ointment	125	Ferndale Laboratories, Inc.
Locoid Topical Lotion	125	Ferndale Laboratories, Inc.
Lodine Capsules	223	Wyeth-Ayerst Laboratories
Lodine Tabs	223	Wyeth-Ayerst Laboratories
Lodine XL Capsules	223	Wyeth-Ayerst Laboratories
Lodine XL Tabs	223	Wyeth-Ayerst Laboratories
Lodosyn	114	Dupont Pharma Company
Lodrane Allergy Capsules	117	ECR Pharmaceuticals
Lodrane LD Capsules	117	ECR Pharmaceuticals
Lodrane Liquid	117	ECR Pharmaceuticals
Loestrin	187	Warner-Lambert
Lopressor	134	Geneva Pharmaceuticals
Lopressor HCT	134	Geneva Pharmaceuticals
Lorabid Pulvules	119	Eli Lilly and Company
Lorabid Suspension	119	Eli Lilly and Company
Lotensin	114	Dupont Pharma Company
Lotensin	134	Geneva Pharmaceuticals
Lotensin	174	Novartis Pharmaceuticals
Lotensin HCT	134	Geneva Pharmaceuticals
Lotensin HCT	174	Novartis Pharmaceuticals
Lotrel	134	Geneva Pharmaceuticals
Lotrel	174	Novartis Pharmaceuticals
Lotrimin Cream	205	Schering Labs/Key Pharm.
Lotrimin Lotion	205	Schering Labs/Key Pharm.
Lotrimin Topical Ointment	205	Schering Labs/Key Pharm.
Lotrisone Cream	205	Schering Labs/Key Pharm.
Lotronex	137	Glaxo Wellcome, Inc.
Lovenox	196	Rhone Poulenc Rorer, Inc.
Loxitane	156	Lederle Labs
Lozol	196	Rhone Poulenc Rorer, Inc.
Ludiomil	134	Geneva Pharmaceuticals
Lupron	216	TAP Pharmaceuticals

MEDICATION	Page	PROGRAM PROVIDER
Lutrepulse	126	Ferring Pharmaceuticals,Inc.
Luvox 25 mg	214	Solvay Pharmaceuticals,Inc.
Luvox 50 mg	214	Solvay Pharmaceuticals,Inc.
Luvox 100 mg	214	Solvay Pharmaceuticals,Inc.
Lysodren	99	Bristol-Myers Access
Macrobid	194	Proctor & Gamble Pharm.
Macrodantin	194	Proctor & Gamble Pharm.
Mag-Ox 400 mg	96	Blaine Company, Inc.
Magnesium Sulfate Injectable	76	AstraZeneca LP, Inc.
Mandol Vials	119	Eli Lilly and Company
Marinol	189	Pfizer Pharmaceutical, Inc.
Marinol	201	Roxane Laboratories, Inc.
Materna	156	Lederle Labs
Matulane	172	NORD
Mavik	155	Knoll Pharmaceutical Co.
Maxair Autohaler	54	3M Pharmaceuticals
Maxair Inhaler	54	3M Pharmaceuticals
Maxalt	163	Merck & Company
Maxzide	94	Bertek Pharmaceuticals,Inc.
Maxzide-25	94	Bertek Pharmaceuticals
Megace Oral Suspension	99	Bristol-Myers Access
Megace Tablets	99	Bristol-Myers Access
Menest 0.3 mg Capsules	168	Monarch Pharmaceuticals
Menest 0.625 mg Capsules	168	Monarch Pharmaceuticals
Menest 1.25 mg Capsules	168	Monarch Pharmaceuticals
Menest 2.5 mg Tabs	168	Monarch Pharmaceuticals
Menomune	172	NORD
Mephyton	163	Merck & Company
Mepron	137	Glaxo Wellcome, Inc.
Mesnex	99	Bristol-Myers Access
Mestinon Injectable	145	ICN Pharmaceuticals
Mestinon Syrup	145	ICN Pharmaceuticals
Mestinon Tablets	145	ICN Pharmaceuticals
Mestinon Timespan Tabs	145	ICN Pharmaceuticals
Metabolic Formulas	159	Mead-Johnson and Co.
Methazolamide	223	Wyeth-Ayerst Laboratories
Methotrexate	223	Wyeth-Ayerst Laboratories

MEDICATION	Page	PROGRAM PROVIDER
Methotrexate Injectable	147	Immunex Corporation
Methotrexate Sodium Tabs	147	Immunex Corporation
Methyldopa	223	Wyeth-Ayerst Laboratories
Meticorten	205	Schering Labs/Key Pharm.
Metopirone Capsules	174	Novartis Pharmaceuticals
MetroCream	130	Galderma Laboratories
Metrodin	210	Serono Laboratories
MetroGel	130	Galderma Laboratories
MetroGel-Vaginal	54	3M Pharmaceuticals
MetroLotion	130	Galderma Laboratories
Mevacor	163	Merck & Company
Mexitil	97	Boehringer Ingelheim
Mezlin	89	Bayer Pharmaceutical
Miacalcin	174	Novartis Pharmaceuticals
Micardis	97	Boehringer Ingelheim
Micronor	180	Ortho-McNeil Pharm.
Midrin	103	Carnrick Laboratories
Migranal Nasal Spray	174	Novartis Pharmaceuticals
Minipress	189	Pfizer Pharmaceutical, Inc.
Minitran Transdermal	54	3M Pharmaceuticals
Minizide	189	Pfizer Pharmaceutical, Inc.
Minocin	223	Wyeth-Ayerst Laboratories
Minocin Capsules	156	Lederle Labs
Minocin Oral Solution	156	Lederle Labs
Mintezol Chewable Tabs	163	Merck & Company
Mintezol Oral Suspension	163	Merck & Company
Miradon	205	Schering Labs/Key Pharm.
Mirapex	192	Pharmacia & Upjohn
Mithracin	89	Bayer Pharmaceutical
Mitrolan	223	Wyeth-Ayerst Laboratories
Mobic	97	Boehringer Ingelheim
Modicon	180	Ortho-McNeil Pharm.
Moduretic	163	Merck & Company
Monistat Derm	180	Ortho-McNeil Pharm.
Monistat-3	180	Ortho-McNeil Pharm.
Monodox	178	Oclassen Dermatologics,Inc.
Monopril	100	Bristol-Myers Foundation

MEDICATION	Page	PROGRAM PROVIDER
Monopril-HCT	100	Bristol-Myers Foundation
Motilium	150	Janssen Pharmaceutica
Motofen	70	Amarin Pharmaceuticals
Motofen	103	Carnrick Laboratories
MRV	89	Bayer Pharmaceutical
MS Contin	195	Purdue Frederick Company
Mucomyst	100	Bristol-Myers Foundation
Mucomyst-10	100	Bristol-Myers Foundation
Mucomyst-20	100	Bristol-Myers Foundation
Mustargen	163	Merck & Company
Mutamycin	99	Bristol-Myers Access
Myanbutol	116	Dura Pharmaceuticals,Inc.
Myanbutol	156	Lederle Labs
Mycelex Triche	67	Alza Pharmaceuticals
Mycobutin	192	Pharmacia & Upjohn
Mycolog II Cream	100	Bristol-Myers Foundation
Mycolog II Lotion	100	Bristol-Myers Foundation
Mycostatin	100	Bristol-Myers Foundation
Mycostatin Oral Suspension	99	Bristol-Myers Access
Mycostatin Tabs	99	Bristol-Myers Access
Mykrox	160	Medeva Pharmaceuticals,Inc.
Myleran	137	Glaxo Wellcome, Inc.
Mysoline Suspension	118	Elan Pharmaceuticals, Inc.
Mysoline Tabs	118	Elan Pharmaceuticals, Inc.
Mytelase	203	Sanofi Pharmaceuticals,Inc.
Nalbuphine Injectable	76	AstraZeneca LP, Inc.
Naldecon Ligui-Gel	100	Bristol-Myers Foundation
Naldecon Pediatric Drops	100	Bristol-Myers Foundation
Naldecon Pediatric Syrup	100	Bristol-Myers Foundation
Naldecon Syrup	100	Bristol-Myers Foundation
Naldecon Tabs	100	Bristol-Myers Foundation
Naloxone HCL Injectable	76	AstraZeneca LP, Inc.
Naprelan	81	Athena Neurosciences
Naprelan	118	Elan Pharmaceuticals, Inc.
Naprosyn	199	Roche Laboratories
Naprosyn Capsules	199	Roche Laboratories
Naproxen	223	Wyeth-Ayerst Laboratories

MEDICATION	Page	PROGRAM PROVIDER
Naqua	205	Schering Labs/Key Pharm.
Nasacort AQ Inhaler	196	Rhone Poulenc Rorer, Inc.
Nasacort AQ Nasal Spray	196	Rhone Poulenc Rorer, Inc.
Nasalide	199	Roche Laboratories
Nasatab LA Tablets	117	ECR Pharmaceuticals
Nasonex Nasal Spray	205	Schering Labs/Key Pharm.
Naturetin	100	Bristol-Myers Foundation
Navane Capsules	189	Pfizer Pharmaceutical, Inc.
Navane Concentrate	189	Pfizer Pharmaceutical, Inc.
Navelbine	137	Glaxo Wellcome, Inc.
Nebupent	71	American Pharmaceuticals
NegGram Caplets	203	Sanofi Pharmaceuticals,Inc.
NegGram Suspension	203	Sanofi Pharmaceuticals,Inc.
Neodecadron Ophthalmic Ointment	163	Merck & Company
Neoral Capsules	176	Novartis (Sandoz) Pharm.
Neoral Capsules	174	Novartis Pharmaceuticals
Neoral Oral Suspension	174	Novartis Pharmaceuticals
Neosar	192	Pharmacia & Upjohn
Neosporin GU	168	Monarch Pharmaceuticals
Neosporin Ophthalmic Ointment	168	Monarch Pharmaceuticals
Neosporin Ophthalmic Solution	168	Monarch Pharmaceuticals
Neostigmine Methylsulfate Inject	76	AstraZeneca LP, Inc.
Neptazane	156	Lederle Labs
Neptazane	223	Wyeth-Ayerst Laboratories
Nesacaine MF Injectable	76	AstraZeneca LP, Inc.
Neupogen (For Injection)	71	Amgen, Inc.
Neurontin	187	Warner-Lambert
Neutra-Phos	67	Alza Pharmaceuticals
Neutrexin	220	U.S. Bioscience, Inc.
Nexium	76	AstraZeneca LP, Inc.
Niacon	219	Upsher-Smith
Nilandron	142	Hoechst Marion Roussel,Inc.
Nimotope	89	Bayer Pharmaceutical
Nistatin Suspension	223	Wyeth-Ayerst Laboratories
Nitrek	94	Bertek Pharmaceuticals,Inc.
Nitro-Dur	154	Key Pharmaceuticals
Nitro-Dur	205	Schering Labs/Key Pharm.

MEDICATION	Page	PROGRAM PROVIDER
Prozac Oral	113	Dista Products
Prozac Pulvules	113	Dista Products
Psorcon .05% Cream	112	Dermik Laboratories
Psorcon .05% Ointment	112	Dermik Laboratories
Psorcon Cream E	112	Dermik Laboratories
Psorcon Ointment E	112	Dermik Laboratories
Pulmocort Respules	79	AstraZeneca Foundation
Pulmozyme	133	Genentech, Inc.
Purinethol	137	Glaxo Wellcome, Inc.
Pyrazinamide	156	Lederle Labs
Pyrazinamide	223	Wyeth-Ayerst Laboratories
Quarzan	199	Roche Laboratories
Questran Light	100	Bristol-Myers Foundation
Questran Oral	100	Bristol-Myers Foundation
Questran Suspension	100	Bristol-Myers Foundation
Quibron	168	Monarch Pharmaceuticals
Quinaglute Dura-Tabs 324 mg	92	Berlex Laboratories
Quinidex Exiler	56	A.H. Robins Co.
Quinidex Extentabs	223	Wyeth-Ayerst Laboratories
Quinidex Tabs	56	A.H. Robins Co.
Quinidine Gluconate	119	Eli Lilly and Company
Quinidine Sulfate	223	Wyeth-Ayerst Laboratories
QVAR Inhaler	54	3M Pharmaceuticals
RabAvert	110	Chiron Therapeutics
Rauzide	100	Bristol-Myers Foundation
Reasec	150	Janssen Pharmaceutica
Rebetron	207	Schering-Plough Oncology
Recombinate	88	Baxter Laboratories
Refresh	66	Allergan Pharmaceuticals,Inc.
Refresh Plus	66	Allergan Pharmaceuticals,Inc.
Refresh PM	66	Allergan Pharmaceuticals,Inc.
Regitine	134	Geneva Pharmaceuticals
Reglan	223	Wyeth-Ayerst Laboratories
Reglan Syrup	56	A.H. Robins Co
Reglan Tabs	56	A.H. Robins Co.
Regranex	150	Janssen Pharmaceutica

MEDICATION	Page	PROGRAM PROVIDER
Robinul	143	Horizon Pharmaceuticals
Robinul Forte	143	Horizon Pharmaceuticals
Robinul Forte Tabs	56	A.H. Robins Co.
Robinul Tabs	56	A.H. Robins Co.
Rocaltrol Capsules	199	Roche Laboratories
Rocaltrol Tabs	199	Roche Laboratories
Rocephin	199	Roche Laboratories
Roferon-A	199	Roche Laboratories
Rowasa Enema	214	Solvay Pharmaceuticals,Inc.
Roxanol	189	Pfizer Pharmaceutical, Inc.
Roxanol 20 ml	201	Roxane Laboratories,Inc.
Roxanol 100	189	Pfizer Pharmaceutical, Inc.
Roxanol 100 Oral Concentrate	201	Roxane Laboratories,Inc.
Roxanol 120 ml	201	Roxane Laboratories,Inc.
Rubex	99	Bristol-Myers Access
Rythmol 150 mg	155	Knoll Pharmaceutical Co.
Rythmol 300 mg	155	Knoll Pharmaceutical Co.
Salagen	167	MGI Pharm., Inc.
Salflex	70	Amarin Pharmaceuticals
Salflex	103	Carnrick Laboratories
Salmex	70	Amarin Pharmaceuticals
Sandimmune	174	Novartis Pharmaceuticals
Sandimmune Capsules	176	Novartis (Sandoz) Pharm.
Sandimmune Oral Suspension	176	Novartis (Sandoz) Pharm.
Sandoglobulin	176	Novartis (Sandoz) Pharm.
Sandostatin	176	Novartis (Sandoz) Pharm.
Sandostatin	174	Novartis Pharmaceuticals
Sandostatin LAR Depot	174	Novartis Pharmaceuticals
ScandiCal	84	Axcan-Scandipharm, Inc.
ScandiShake	84	Axcan-Scandipharm, Inc.
Sebizon	205	Schering Labs/Key Pharm.
Secretin-Ferring	126	Ferring Pharmaceuticals,Inc.
Sectral	223	Wyeth-Ayerst Laboratories
Selegiline	223	Wyeth-Ayerst Laboratories
Semap	150	Janssen Pharmaceutica
Semprex-D	160	Medeva Pharmaceuticals,Inc.

MEDICATION	Page	PROGRAM PROVIDER
Targretin Gel	157	Ligard Pharmaceuticals
Tarka	155	Knoll Pharmaceutical Co.
Tasmar	199	Roche Laboratories
Taxol	99	Bristol-Myers Access
Taxotere	83	Aventis-Oncology Pact Prg.
Taxotere	197	Rhone Poulenc Rorer, Inc.
Tears Plus	66	Allergan Pharmaceuticals,Inc.
Tegretol XR Tabs	174	Novartis Pharmaceuticals
Tegretol Chewable Tabs	134	Geneva Pharmaceuticals
Tegretol Chewable Tabs	174	Novartis Pharmaceuticals
Tegretol Oral Suspension	174	Novartis Pharmaceuticals
Tegretol PM Capsules	134	Geneva Pharmaceuticals
Tegretol PM Capsules	174	Novartis Pharmaceuticals
Tegretol Suspension	134	Geneva Pharmaceuticals
Tegretol Tabs	134	Geneva Pharmaceuticals
Tegretol XR Tabs	134	Geneva Pharmaceuticals
Temodar	207	Schering-Plough Oncology
Temovate Cream	137	Glaxo Wellcome, Inc.
Temovate E Enollient	137	Glaxo Wellcome, Inc.
Temovate Lotion	137	Glaxo Wellcome, Inc.
Temovate Ointment	137	Glaxo Wellcome, Inc.
Temovate Scalp Application	137	Glaxo Wellcome, Inc.
Tenex	56	A.H. Robins Co.
Tenex	223	Wyeth-Ayerst Laboratories
Tenoretic	79	AstraZeneca Foundation
Tenormin Tabs	79	AstraZeneca Foundation
Tensilon Injectable	144	ICN Pharmaceuticals, Inc.
Tequin	100	Bristol-Myers Foundation
Terazol	180	Ortho-McNeil Pharm.
Teslac	99	Bristol-Myers Access
Tessalon Perls	127	Forest Pharmaceuticals,Inc.
Testoderm Transdermal	67	Alza Pharmaceuticals
Tetracycline	223	Wyeth-Ayerst Laboratories
Thalitone 15 mg Tabs	168	Monarch Pharmaceuticals
Thalitone 25 mg Tabs	168	Monarch Pharmaceuticals
Thalomid	105	Celgene Corporation

MEDICATION	Page	PROGRAM PROVIDER
Vanoxide-HC Lotion	112	Dermik Laboratories
Vascor	180	Ortho-McNeil Pharm.
Vasodilan	100	Bristol-Myers Foundation
Vaseretic	163	Merck & Company
Vasotec	163	Merck & Company
Vasoxyl	137	Glaxo Wellcome, Inc.
Velban	119	Eli Lilly and Company
Velosulin BR	177	Novo-Nordisk Pharm.,Inc.
Velstar Intravesical Solution	160	Medeva Pharmaceuticals,Inc.
Venomil Maintenance	89	Bayer Pharmaceutical
Ventolin	137	Glaxo Wellcome, Inc.
VePesid	99	Bristol-Myers Access
Vermox	150	Janssen Pharmaceutica
Vesanoid	199	Roche Laboratories
Viagra	189	Pfizer Pharmaceutical, Inc.
Vibra-Tabs	189	Pfizer Pharmaceutical, Inc.
Vibramycin	189	Pfizer Pharmaceutical, Inc.
Videx Pediatric Oral Powder	99	Bristol-Myers Access
Videx Oral Suspension	99	Bristol-Myers Access
Vincsar PFS	192	Pharmacia & Upjohn
Viokase	184	Paddock Laboratories, Inc.
Viokase Powder	87	Axcan-Scandipharm, Inc.
Viokase Tabs	87	Axcan-Scandipharm, Inc.
Vioxx	163	Merck & Company
Vira-A Ophthalmic Ointment	168	Monarch Pharmaceuticals
Viracept	62	Agouron Pharmaceuticals
Viramune	189	Pfizer Pharmaceutical, Inc.
Viramune Oral Suspension	201	Roxane Laboratories,Inc.
Virazole	144	ICN Pharmaceuticals, Inc.
Viroptic 1% Ophthalmic Solution	168	Monarch Pharmaceuticals
Vistaril Capsules	189	Pfizer Pharmaceutical, Inc.
Vistaril Oral Concentrate	189	Pfizer Pharmaceutical, Inc.
Vistaril Tabs	189	Pfizer Pharmaceutical, Inc.
Vistide	136	Gilead Science Corp.
Vitadye Lotion	144	ICN Pharmaceuticals, Inc.
Vivactil	163	Merck & Company

ALPHABETICAL LISTING

OF

ASSISTANCE PROGRAMS

COMPANY: 3M Pharmaceuticals

PROGRAM ADDRESS: Medical Services Department
3M Center Bldg, 275-2E-13
P.O. Box 33275
St. Paul, MN 55133-3275

TOLL FREE PHONE NUMBER: 800-328-0255
ALTERNATIVE NUMBER: 651-736-4930
FAX NUMBER: 651-733-6068

ELIGIBILITY: You cannot have insurance that provides prescription coverage and you must be ineligible for State Medicaid. The physician should agree that your income is so low that purchasing the medication will cause a hardship.

ENROLLMENT: The doctor's office or a social worker must call 3M's Medical Services Department for the enrollment application. 3M will ask for the name of the patient, the name of the doctor, the doctor's address, phone number, and the name of the medication requested.

FROM YOUR DOCTOR: The application is patient-specific and is sent to your doctor with all the information on it except for the doctor's signature and DEA number. A prescription is not needed. Your doctor will complete the application; sign the application, and mail it to 3M's Medical Services Department.

WHAT YOU HAVE TO DO: Stay in contact with your doctor's office. You must provide the necessary financial information and sign the form.

WHERE THE MEDICATION GOES: The medication will be sent to your doctor's office. The medication will not be sent to a P.O. Box.

AMOUNT GIVEN AT ONE TIME: Usually three (3) month supply, but varies according to the medication.

NO. OF REFILLS: Indefinite (except for Aldar (2 boxes/8 weeks) and MetroGel (one-time shipment). You may call in repeat orders.

GENERAL INFORMATION: You can call between 9:00 am and 4:00 pm, Central Time, Monday through Friday.

Special phone numbers to use for specific medications:

Aldara Cream 5%: 800-814-1795

MEDICATIONS AVAILABLE: Aldara Crème 5%, Alu-Cap, Alu-Tab, Disalcid Cap, Disalcid Tabs, Maxair Autohaler, Maxair Inhaler, MetroGel-Vaginal, Minitran Transdermal, Norflex ER Tabs, Norflex Injection, Norgesic Forte, Norgesic Tabs, QVAR Inhaler, Tambocor, Theolair SR, Theolair Tablets

COMPANY: A.H. Robins Company

PROGRAM ADDRESS: A.H. Robins Company
                        1407 Cummings Drive
                        Richmond, VA 23220

TOLL FREE PHONE NUMBER: 800-934-5556
ALTERNATIVE NUMBER: 610-688-4400

ELIGIBILITY: You cannot have insurance that provides prescription coverage and you must be ineligible for State Medicaid.

ENROLLMENT: Anyone can call for an enrollment application.

FROM YOUR DOCTOR: Your doctor will complete the application, attach a prescription (if necessary), sign the application, and mail it to Wyeth-Ayerst.

WHAT YOU HAVE TO DO: Stay in contact with your doctor's office. Your signature is required.

WHERE THE MEDICATION GOES: The medication will be sent to your doctor's office. The medication will not be sent to a P.O. Box.

AMOUNT GIVEN AT ONE TIME: A 90-day supply.

TIME TO GET MEDICATION: Approximately 4-5 weeks.

GENERAL INFORMATION: You can call between 9:00 am and 4:00 pm, Eastern Time, Monday through Friday.

MEDICATIONS AVAILABLE: Donnazyme, Quinidex Exiler, Quinidex Tabs, Reglan Syrup, Reglan Tabs, Robaxin Tabs, Robaxin 750 Tabs, Robaxisal, Robinul Forte Tabs, Robinul Tabs, Tenex

COMPANY: Abbott Laboratories
Pharmaceutical Products Division

PROGRAM ADDRESS: Abbott Laboratories
Dept. 31C, AP-30
100 Abbott Park Rd.
Abbott Park, IL 60064

TOLL FREE PHONE NUMBER: 800-255-5162

ELIGIBILITY: You cannot have insurance that provides prescription coverage and you must be ineligible for State Medicaid. Your income must fall between 100-200% (see pg. 249-250) of the Federal Poverty Guideline. If you don't fall within these guidelines, then a letter of rejection from Medicaid is required.

ENROLLMENT: The doctor's office must call for the enrollment application. Basic information is required when the application is requested. It should arrive in about two weeks.

FROM YOUR DOCTOR: Your doctor will complete the application, attach a prescription (if required), sign the application, and mail it to Abbott Laboratories, Pharmaceutical Products Division.

WHAT YOU HAVE TO DO: Stay in contact with your doctor's office. Detailed financial and insurance information is required. Proof of your income may be requested. Your signature is required.

WHERE THE MEDICATION GOES: The medication will be sent to your doctor's office. The medication will not be sent to a P.O. Box.

AMOUNT GIVEN AT ONE TIME: A 30-day supply is sent, followed by three (3) 90-day supplies. Call your doctor when your supply is getting low.

NO. OF REFILLS: After 10-12 months, you will need to call and request a re-application form.

GENERAL INFORMATION: You can call between 8:30 am and 4:30 pm, Central Time, Monday through Friday.

MEDICATIONS AVAILABLE: Depakote Capsules, Depakote Sprinkle Capsules, Depakote Syrup, Depakote Tabs, Gabitril

COMPANY: Abbott Laboratories

PROGRAM ADDRESS: Abbott Biaxin Patient Assistance Program
                            Parexel/S&FA
                            1101 King St., Suite 600
                            Alexandria, VA 22314

TOLL FREE PHONE NUMBER: 800-688-9118
ALTERNATIVE NUMBER: 800-255-5162

ELIGIBILITY: You cannot have insurance that provides prescription coverage and you must be ineligible for State Medicaid. You must not be eligible for help through the Ryan White Funding Program or any government assistance program.

ENROLLMENT: Your doctor's office should call for the enrollment application. The enrollment form is sent to your doctor.

FROM YOUR DOCTOR: Your doctor will complete the application, attach a prescription (if necessary), sign the application, and mail it to Abbott Biaxin Patient Assistance Program. Your doctor must provide a CD-4 cell count lab results.

WHAT YOU HAVE TO DO: Stay in contact with your doctor's office. You must provide detailed financial and insurance information, proof of your income and your household income is required.

WHERE THE MEDICATION GOES: The medication will be sent to your doctor's office. The medication will not be sent to a P.O. Box.

AMOUNT GIVEN AT ONE TIME: 180 tablets (depends on dosing) for 90-day period. Your doctor needs to write a letter if the dosing is more than recommended.

TIME TO GET MEDICATION: Usually within 2-3 weeks.

NO. OF REFILLS: Use a new application, but no CD-4 level is required.

GENERAL INFORMATION: You can call between 8:30 am and 5:30 pm, Eastern Time, Monday through Friday. Biaxin AIDS patient assistance program is for patients with micro-bacterial infections or for prophylactic use. The CD-4 count must be below 100 to qualify. Biaxin is no longer available for Non-AIDS patients.

MEDICATIONS AVAILABLE: Biaxin Oral Suspension, Biaxin Tabs

COMPANY: Abbott Laboratories

PROGRAM ADDRESS: NORTAP
490 Second Street, Suite 201
San Francisco, CA 94107

TOLL FREE PHONE NUMBER: 800-659-9050

ELIGIBILITY: You cannot have insurance that provides prescription coverage and you must be ineligible for State Medicaid. The income guideline for the program is 200% (see pg. 249-250) of the Federal Poverty Guideline.

ENROLLMENT: Your doctor's office must call for the enrollment application and registration.

FROM YOUR DOCTOR: Your doctor's office must make the request for program participation before the application will be sent. The application is sent to your doctor's office. Your doctor will complete the application, attach a prescription (if necessary), sign the application, and mail it to NORTAP.

WHAT YOU HAVE TO DO: Stay in contact with your doctor's office. The company requires detailed financial and insurance information, including proof of your income and your total household income.

WHERE THE MEDICATION GOES: The medication will be sent to your doctor's office. The medication will not be sent to a P.O. Box.

AMOUNT GIVEN AT ONE TIME: Enough for 9-1/2 months.

GENERAL INFORMATION: If your state AIDS assistance program covers this drug, then, in order to qualify, you will need a letter of denial from your state. If your state's guidelines are lower than that and you are somewhere in between, then you probably are eligible. You can call between 9:00 am and 4:00 pm, Pacific Time, Monday through Friday.

MEDICATION AVAILABLE: Norvir Oral Suspension

COMPANY: Agouron Pharmaceuticals, Inc.

PROGRAM ADDRESS: Agouron Pharmaceuticals, Inc.
                        10350 North Torrey Pines Rd.
                        La Jolla, CA 92037-1020

TOLL FREE PHONE NUMBER: 888-777-6637

ELIGIBILITY: You cannot have insurance that provides prescription coverage and you must be ineligible for State Medicaid. Income guidelines are 150% (see pg. 249-250) of the Federal Poverty Guideline, but they will also consider other medical expenses.

ENROLLMENT: Anyone can call to start the enrollment process with the patient's permission but it may be best to have your doctor's office call. They will need the doctor's name, DEA number, street address, and phone number. They will need your name, phone number, social security number, birth date, number of people in the household, number of dependents, and annual income. The application is mailed to your doctor.

FROM YOUR DOCTOR: Your doctor will complete the first page of the application, including your most recent CD-4 count and viral load, attach a prescription if a four-month supply of the medicine is required, sign the application, and mail it to Agouron Pharmaceuticals, Inc.

WHAT YOU HAVE TO DO: Stay in contact with your doctor's office. You will have to provide detailed financial and insurance information, although some of the information is optional. Your signature is required.

WHERE THE MEDICATION GOES: The medication will be sent to your doctor's office. The medication will not be sent to a P.O. Box.

AMOUNT GIVEN AT ONE TIME: A three-weeks' supply is sent for a four-month period.

NO. OF REFILLS: When the last shipment is sent, the doctor is sent a postcard prompting the doctor to call if you need to reapply.

GENERAL INFORMATION: You can call between 9:00 am and 4:00 pm, Pacific Time, Monday through Friday.

MEDICATION AVAILABLE: Viracept

COMPANY: Alcon Labs

PROGRAM ADDRESS: Needy Patient Program
         Attn S2-7
         6201 S. Freeway
         Ft. Worth, TX 76134

TOLL FREE PHONE NUMBER: 800-451-3937
ALTERNATIVE NUMBER: 817-298-0450

ELIGIBILITY: You cannot have insurance that provides prescription coverage and you must be ineligible for State Medicaid.

ENROLLMENT: There is no formal application. Your doctor's office should call.

FROM YOUR DOCTOR: Your doctor will send in a prescription with their DEA number, license number, address, a brief note saying you can't afford the medication, and mail it to Needy Patient Program.

WHAT YOU HAVE TO DO: Stay in contact with your doctor's office. You need to let your doctor know one month before running out of the medicine.

WHERE THE MEDICATION GOES: The medication will be sent to your doctor's office. The medication will not be sent to a P.O. Box.

AMOUNT GIVEN AT ONE TIME: The number depends on the medicine.

GENERAL INFORMATION: You can call between 9:00 am and 5:00 pm, Central Time, Monday through Friday.

MEDICATIONS AVAILABLE: Azopt Oral Suspension, Betoptic S Ophthalmic Suspension, Glacon, Isopto Carbachol, Isopto Carpine, Isopto Cetapred, Isopto Homatropine, Isopto Hyoscine, Iopidine Ophthalmic Suspension, Pilopine HS

COMPANY: Allergan, Inc.

PROGRAM ADDRESS: Botox Patient Assistance Program
                       Allergan, Inc.
                       2525 Dupont Dr.
                       Irvine, CA 92713

TOLL FREE PHONE NUMBER: 800-347-4500
ALTERNATIVE NUMBER: 714-752-4500
FAX NUMBER: 714-955-6976

ELIGIBILITY: You cannot have insurance that provides prescription coverage and you must be ineligible for State Medicaid.

ENROLLMENT: You doctor's office must calls for the enrollment application, which are sent to the doctor's office.

FROM YOUR DOCTOR: Doctor has to agree to waive the office visit fee. Your doctor will complete the application, attach a prescription (if necessary), sign the application, and mail it to Botox Patient Assistance Program.

WHAT YOU HAVE TO DO: Stay in contact with your doctor's office. You will have to provide detailed financial and insurance information

WHERE THE MEDICATION GOES: The medication will be sent to your doctor's office. The medication will not be sent to a P.O. Box.

AMOUNT GIVEN AT ONE TIME: Usually a 90-day supply.

GENERAL INFORMATION: You can call between 9:00 am and 4:00 pm, Pacific Time, Monday through Friday.

MEDICATION AVAILABLE: Botox

COMPANY: Allergan Pharmaceuticals, Inc.

PROGRAM ADDRESS: Patient Assistance Program
                            c/o Physician Services (T1-2G)
                            2525 Dupont Drive.
                            P O Box 19534
                            Irvine, CA 92623-95534

TOLL FREE PHONE NUMBER: 800-347-4500

ELIGIBILITY: You cannot have insurance that provides prescription coverage and you must be ineligible for State Medicaid. Your household income, for a family of one (1), must be less than $12,000 a year. Your household income, for a family of two (2), must be less than $18,000 a year.

ENROLLMENT: Anyone can call for the enrollment application. Registration is done by phone. The form is sent only to the ophthalmologists or optometrists.

FROM YOUR DOCTOR: Your doctor will complete the application, including DEA number, attach a prescription (if necessary), sign the application (it must be an original signature), including DEA number and mail it to Patient Assistance Program. Your doctor may send on office stationery a letter including the date of the request, state license number, your name, address, phone number, name of product, strength and size.

WHAT YOU HAVE TO DO: Stay in contact with your doctor's office.

WHERE THE MEDICATION GOES: The medication will be sent to your doctor's office. The medication will not be sent to a P.O. Box. Over-the-counter medications may be sent directly to you if so requested and if your address is sent with the request.

GENERAL INFORMATION: You can call between 9:00 am and 4:00 pm, Pacific Time, Monday through Friday.

MEDICATIONS AVAILABLE: Alphagan Ophthalmic Suspension, Betagan Ophthalmic Suspension, Celluvisc Lubricant Eye Drops, Epifrin Ophthalmic Suspension, Lacri-Lube, Pilagan, Propine Ophthalmic Suspension, Refresh, Refresh Plus, Refresh PM, Tears Plus

COMPANY: Alza Pharmaceuticals

PROGRAM ADDRESS: Alza Indigent Patient Assistance Program
C/O CRC, Inc.
8990 Springbrook Drive
Minneapolis, MN 55433

TOLL FREE PHONE NUMBER: 800-577-3788
ALTERNATIVE NUMBER: 415-962-4297

ELIGIBILITY: You cannot have insurance that provides prescription coverage and you must be ineligible for State Medicaid.

ENROLLMENT: The doctor's office must call to register you. Then the company will send a patient-specific/doctor-specific enrollment application.

FROM YOUR DOCTOR: Your doctor will complete the application, attach a prescription (if necessary), send diagnostic and treatment information, sign the application, and mail it to Alza Indigent Patient Assistance Program.

WHAT YOU HAVE TO DO: Stay in contact with your doctor's office. You will have to provide detailed financial and insurance information. You must sign the form.

WHERE THE MEDICATION GOES: The medication will be sent to your doctor's office. The medication will not be sent to a P.O. Box.

AMOUNT GIVEN AT ONE TIME: Usually a 90-day supply.

NO. OF REFILLS: The doctor calls and the company will send a product request card. A new application is needed once a year.

GENERAL INFORMATION: This program is run by Comprehensive Reimbursement Consultants. The forms are non-transferable and are patient-specific. You can call between 9:00 am and 4:00 pm, Central Time, Monday through Friday.

MEDICATIONS AVAILABLE: Bicitra, Ditropan Tabs, Ditropan Syrup, Ditropan XL, Doxil Injectable, Elmiron Caps, Ethyol (for Injection), Mycelex Triche, Neutra-Phos, Ocusert, PolyCitra LC Syrup, PolyCitra Syrup, PolyCitra-K Crystals, PolyCitra-K Oral Suspension, Progestasert, Testoderm Transdermal, Urispas

COMPANY: Alza Pharmaceuticals

PROGRAM ADDRESS: Alza Oncology Connection Program
c/o Documedics
1250 Bayhill Drive
Suite 300
San Bruno, CA 94066

TOLL FREE PHONE NUMBER: 800-482-1083

ELIGIBILITY: You cannot have insurance that provides prescription coverage and you must be ineligible for State Medicaid.

ENROLLMENT: Your doctor's office must call for the enrollment application. The company will fax the information and application to your doctor.

FROM YOUR DOCTOR: Your doctor will complete the application, attach a prescription (if necessary), sign the application, and mail it to Alza Oncology Connection Program. Your doctor will have to state whether you are on chemo or radiation and the names of any oral medications you are taking.

WHAT YOU HAVE TO DO: Stay in contact with your doctor's office. You will have to provide financial and insurance information.

WHERE THE MEDICATION GOES: The medication will be sent to your doctor's office. The medication will not be sent to a P.O. Box.

AMOUNT GIVEN AT ONE TIME: Depends on the medication.

GENERAL INFORMATION: You can call between 9:00 am and 4:00 pm, Pacific Time, Monday through Friday.

MEDICATIONS AVAILABLE: Doxil Injectable, Ethyol (for Injection),

COMPANY: Amarin Pharmaceuticals

PROGRAM ADDRESS: Amarin Pharmaceuticals
                          Indigent Patient Program
                          25 Independence Boulevard
                          Warren, NJ 07059

TOLL FREE PHONE NUMBER: 908-580-5535
FAX NUMBER: 908-580-9390

ELIGIBILITY: You cannot have insurance that provides prescription coverage and you must be ineligible for State Medicaid.

ENROLLMENT: Your doctor's office must call for an enrollment application form.

FROM YOUR DOCTOR: Your doctor will complete the application, attach a prescription including the doctor's state license number on prescription, sign the application, and mail it to Amarin Pharmaceuticals. The enrollment application and prescription can be faxed back, unless it is for a controlled substance. Then the enrollment application and prescription must be mailed.

WHAT YOU HAVE TO DO: Stay in contact with your doctor's office.

WHERE THE MEDICATION GOES: The medication will be sent to your doctor's office. The medication will not be sent to a P.O. Box.

AMOUNT GIVEN AT ONE TIME: Usually a 90-day supply.

GENERAL INFORMATION: Bontril will only be available to morbidly obese or otherwise high-risk patients. Exgest is only available in stock bottles. You can call between 9:00 am and 4:00 pm, Eastern Time, Monday through Friday.

MEDICATIONS AVAILABLE: Bontril, Capital Oral Suspension, Codeine Oral Suspension, Exgest, Hydrocet, Motofen, Nolahist, Nolamine, Phrenilin, Phrenilin Forte, Salflex, Salmex

COMPANY: American Pharmaceuticals

PROGRAM ADDRESS: Nebupent Patient Assistance Program
                       1101 Perimeter Drive, Suite 300
                       Schaumberg, IL 60173

PHONE NUMBER: 847-330-1289

ELIGIBILITY: You cannot have insurance that provides prescription coverage and you must be ineligible for State Medicaid.

ENROLLMENT: You doctor's office must call for the enrollment application.

FROM YOUR DOCTOR: Your doctor will complete the application, attach a prescription (if necessary), sign the application, and mail it to Nebupent Patient Assistance Program. Your doctor needs to write a letter on their letterhead including: your financial and insurance information, the name and dose of the drugs needed, their state license number, DEA number, a complete shipping address, and the name of whoever will administer the product. The doctor must sign the letter. The doctor will receive and must sign a contract affirming that the product will not be resold or diverted to another patient

WHAT YOU HAVE TO DO: Inform your doctor of this program and stay in contact with your doctor's office.

WHERE THE MEDICATION GOES: The medicine is sent to whoever will be administer the medication.

AMOUNT GIVEN AT ONE TIME: One course of the medicine, usually a 6-month supply.

NO. OF REFILLS: You have to reapply.

GENERAL INFORMATION: You can call between 9:00 am and 4:00 pm, Central Time, Monday through Friday.

MEDICATION AVAILABLE: Nebupent

COMPANY: Amgen, Inc.

PROGRAM ADDRESS: Amgen Safety Net Program
                          1840 Devavilland Drive
                          Thousand Oaks, CA 91230-1789

TOLL FREE PHONE NUMBER: 800-272-9376
ALTERNATIVE NUMBER: 202-637-6698
FAX NUMBER: 800-282-6436

ELIGIBILITY: You cannot have insurance that provides prescription coverage and you must be ineligible for State Medicaid.

ENROLLMENT: Anyone can for the enrollment. Registration is done by phone. The caller must have your name, Social Security Number, annual family income, insurance information, and average monthly dose of the drug.

FROM YOUR DOCTOR: Your doctor will complete the application, attach a prescription (if necessary), sign the application, and mail it to Amgen Safety Net Program.

WHAT YOU HAVE TO DO: Stay in contact with your doctor's office. You will have to provide detailed financial and insurance information. You must sign the application form

WHERE THE MEDICATION GOES: The medication will be sent to your doctor's office. The medication will not be sent to a P.O. Box. Replacement product provided to the hospital or doctor.

AMOUNT GIVEN AT ONE TIME: Usually a 90-day supply.

NO. OF REFILLS: Up to a 12-month supply.

GENERAL INFORMATION: You can call between 9:00 am and 5:00 pm, Eastern Time, Monday through Friday.

MEDICATIONS AVAILABLE: Epogen, Neupogen

COMPANY: Amgen, Inc.

PROGRAM ADDRESS: Amgen Safety Net Program for Infergen
c/o Medical Technology Hotline
P.O. Box 7710
Washington DC 20044-7710

TOLL FREE PHONE NUMBER: 888-508-8088

ELIGIBILITY: You cannot have insurance that provides prescription coverage and you must be ineligible for State Medicaid.

ENROLLMENT: Anyone can call for the enrollment application. They will have to have your name, Social Security Number, annual family income, insurance information, and the average monthly dose of the medication.

FROM YOUR DOCTOR: Your doctor will complete the application, attach a prescription (if necessary), submit an Infergen Dosage Tracking Form, sign the application, and mail it to Amgen Safety Net Program for Infergen. The sponsorship form needs to be completed only once by a provider. It indicates the provider's understanding of the program and their agreement to comply with its terms.

WHAT YOU HAVE TO DO: Stay in contact with your doctor's office. You will have to provide detailed financial and insurance information. You may be required to send documented proof.

WHERE THE MEDICATION GOES: The medication will be sent to your doctor's office. The medication will not be sent to a P.O. Box.

AMOUNT GIVEN AT ONE TIME: Boxes of Infergen will arrive 3-5 business days after the Infergen Dosage Tracking Form and prescription are received.

NO. OF REFILLS: Enrollment form is good for a year.

GENERAL INFORMATION: You can call between 9:00 am and 5:00 pm, Eastern Time, Monday through Friday. This program is for patients being treated for Hepatitis C.

MEDICATION AVAILABLE: Infergen

COMPANY: Apothecon-Bristol-Myers-Squibb

PROGRAM ADDRESS: Apothecon-Bristol-Myers-Squibb
                           P.O. Box 4500
                           Princeton, NJ 08543-4500

TOLL FREE PHONE NUMBER: 800-437-0994
ALTERNATIVE NUMBER: 800-332-2056

ELIGIBILITY: You cannot have insurance that provides prescription coverage and you must be ineligible for State Medicaid.

ENROLLMENT: Anyone can call for the enrollment application.

FROM YOUR DOCTOR: Your doctor will complete the application, attach a prescription (if necessary), sign the application, and mail it to Apothecon-Bristol-Myers-Squibb.

WHAT YOU HAVE TO DO: Stay in contact with your doctor's office.

WHERE THE MEDICATION GOES: The medication will be sent to your doctor's office. The medication will not be sent to a P.O. Box.

GENERAL INFORMATION: You can call between 9:00 am and 4:00 pm, Eastern Time, Monday through Friday.

MEDICATIONS AVAILABLE: Atenolol, Cephalexin, Cephalexin Oral Suspension, Deseryl, Deseryl Dividose, Fungizone, Penicillin

COMPANY: Astra Merck

PROGRAM ADDRESS: Astra Merck
                        The Fulfillment Center
                        1 Phoenix Center
                        Lincoln Park, NJ 07035

TOLL FREE PHONE NUMBER: 800-355-6044
ALTERNATIVE NUMBER: 800-236-9933

ELIGIBILITY: You cannot have insurance that provides prescription coverage and you must be ineligible for State Medicaid.

ENROLLMENT: Your doctor's office should call for an enrollment application form.

FROM YOUR DOCTOR: Your doctor will complete the application, attach a prescription (if necessary), sign the application, and mail it to Astra Merck.

WHAT YOU HAVE TO DO: Stay in contact with your doctor's office.

WHERE THE MEDICATION GOES: The medication will be sent to your doctor's office. The medication will not be sent to a P.O. Box.

AMOUNT GIVEN AT ONE TIME: Usually a 90-day supply.

GENERAL INFORMATION: You can call between 8:00 am and 5:00 pm, Eastern Time, Monday through Friday.

MEDICATIONS AVAILABLE: Lexxell, Plendil ER, Prilosec DR Caps, Tonocard

COMPANY: AstraZeneca LP, Inc.

PROGRAM ADDRESS: The Fulfillment Center
                        50 Otis St.
                        Westborough, MA 01581-4500

TOLL FREE PHONE NUMBER: 800-355-6044

ELIGIBILITY: You cannot have insurance that provides prescription coverage and you must be ineligible for State Medicaid.

ENROLLMENT: Anyone can call for enrollment application. Ask for the product manager for the medication you need.

FROM YOUR DOCTOR: Your doctor will complete the application, attach a prescription (if necessary), sign the application, and mail it to The Fulfillment Center.

WHAT YOU HAVE TO DO: Stay in contact with your doctor's office. You will need to provide insurance and income information.

WHERE THE MEDICATION GOES: The medication will be sent to your doctor's office. The medication will not be sent to a P.O. Box.

AMOUNT GIVEN AT ONE TIME: Usually a 90-day supply

GENERAL INFORMATION: You can call between 9:00 am and 4:00 pm, Eastern Time, Monday through Friday.

MEDICATIONS AVAILABLE: Atacand, Calcitonin Injectable, Calcium Chloride Injectable, Clindamycin Injectable, Dalgan Injectable, Dobutamine Injectable, Doxorubicin Injectable, Droperidol Injectable, Fentanyl Citrate Injectable, EMLA Cream, EMLA Anesthetic Discs, Etoposide Injectable, Levothyroxine Injectable, Lexxell, Magnesium Sulfate Injectable, Nalbuphine Injectable, Naloxone HCL Injectable, Neostigmine Methylsulfate Injectable, Nesacaine MF Injectable, Nexium, Pancuronium Bromide Injectable, Plendil ER, Polocaine MF Injectable, Prilosec DR, Rhinocort Nasal Inhaler, Sensorcaine Injectable, Sensorcaine Injectable with Epinephrine, Tonocard, Toprol XL Tabs, Xylocaine

COMPANY: AstraZeneca, Inc.

PROGRAM ADDRESS: FAIR Program
                        Reimbursement Division
                        1101 King St., Suite 600
                        Alexandria, VA 22314

TOLL FREE PHONE NUMBER: 800-488-3247
ALTERNATIVE NUMBER: 705-535-5080
FAX NUMBER: 703-683-2239

ELIGIBILITY: You cannot have insurance that provides prescription coverage and you must be ineligible for State Medicaid. You must be newly diagnosed with CMV Retinitis (or have a medical reason for switching to Foscavir from Ganciclovir).

ENROLLMENT: Your doctor's office must call for the enrollment application.

FROM YOUR DOCTOR: Your doctor will complete the application, attach a prescription (if necessary), sign the application, and mail it to FAIR Program.

WHAT YOU HAVE TO DO: Stay in contact with your doctor's office.

WHERE THE MEDICATION GOES: The medication will be sent to your doctor's office. The medication will not be sent to a P.O. Box.

AMOUNT GIVEN AT ONE TIME: Two (2) cases of induction and one (1) case of maintenance, enough for 3 months.

NO. OF REFILLS: Call to say you need to re-enroll.

GENERAL INFORMATION: They keep abreast of policy changes and help to advocate for third-party reimbursement. They can save providers time by researching and clarifying insurance coverage options. Call 800-488-3247 for verification of patient's insurance coverage for Foscavir. You can call between 9:00 am and 4:00 pm, Eastern Time, Monday through Friday.

MEDICATION AVAILABLE: Foscavir

COMPANY: AstraZeneca, Inc.

PROGRAM ADDRESS: AstraZeneca PAP Foundation
                      Patient Assistant Program
                      P.O. Box 15197
                      Wilmington, DE 19850-5197

TOLL FREE PHONE NUMBER: 800-424-3727
ALTERNATIVE NUMBER: 800-698-0085

ELIGIBILITY: You cannot have insurance that provides prescription coverage and you must be ineligible for State Medicaid.

ENROLLMENT: Anyone can call for an enrollment application form. When completing the enrollment application, make sure no questions are left unanswered. If the question doesn't apply, **write "NA" or a similar term.** They will return applications that contain blanks. The form will have your name on it, so it can't be copied.

FROM YOUR DOCTOR: Your doctor will complete the application, sign the application, and mail it to AstraZeneca Foundation PAP. Do not send prescription with application. A prescription is not needed until you are approved for the program.

WHAT YOU HAVE TO DO: Stay in contact with your doctor's office. You will have to provide detailed financial and insurance. Your signature is required. You will need to send the prescription in the provided mailer.

WHERE THE MEDICATION GOES: AstraZeneca Foundation PAP utilizes Express Scripts (mail order pharmacy). Upon approval, an Express Scripts mailer will be sent to you. Place the prescription, a $5.00 money order **(DO NOT SEND CASH)**, and mail it to Express Scripts. The mailers are sent in with a prescription for a three-month supply. Federal Express will deliver the medicines directly to your home. The medication will not be sent to a P.O. Box.

AMOUNT GIVEN AT ONE TIME: Prescriptions must be written for a three-month, 100-day supply. All bottles contain 100 tablets except for Accolate (60 per bottle) and Arimidex (30 per bottle).

GENERAL INFORMATION: You can call between 9:00 am and 4:00 pm, Eastern Time, Monday through Friday.

Zoladex requires additional approval from the company and prescriptions must be written for one dose of 3.6 mg depot or 1 dose of 10.8 mg depot. Prescriptions for more than one depot can't be honored.

MEDICATIONS AVAILABLE: Accolate, Arimidex, Casodex, Nolvadex, Pulmocort Respules, Seroquel, Sular, Sorbitrate Tabs, Sorbitrate Chewable Tabs, Tenoretic, Tenormin Tabs, Zestoretic, Zestril, Zoladex, Zomig

COMPANY: Athena Neurosciences

PROGRAM ADDRESS: Prescription Assistance Program
c/o Athena Rx Home Pharmacy
800 Gateway Blvd.
South San Francisco, CA 94080

TOLL FREE PHONE NUMBER: 800-621-4835 ext 7788
ALTERNATIVE NUMBER: 888-638-7605, 800-578-7977
FAX NUMBER: 800-528-5256

ELIGIBILITY: You cannot have insurance that provides prescription coverage; you must be ineligible for State Medicaid, provide a letter of denial from the State Medicaid program, and send copies of your most recent tax return or three consecutive bank statements if you don't file taxes. Your net worth must be less than $30,000.

ENROLLMENT: Anyone can call to enroll you. They will have to have your name, address, phone number, Social Security Number, insurance information, income information, and your net worth.

FROM YOUR DOCTOR: Your doctor will complete the application. On their letterhead: They must include your name, address, phone, social security number, and your date of birth. The doctor's DEA number, state license, stating you have a net worth less than $30,000, attach a prescription (if necessary), sign the application, and mail it to Prescription Assistance Program Prescription. The letter and prescription can be faxed to above number only by a doctor's office, or the application and prescription can be mailed by anyone.

WHAT YOU HAVE TO DO: Stay in contact with your doctor's office.

WHERE THE MEDICATION GOES: Upon approval, the company contacts you, sets up pharmacy records and ships product directly to you via UPS Ground (2-7 work days). The medication will not be sent to a P.O. Box.

AMOUNT GIVEN AT ONE TIME: Usually a 90-day supply.

GENERAL INFORMATION: You must be U.S. resident. You can call between 9:00 am and 4:00 pm, Pacific Time, Monday through Friday.

MEDICATIONS AVAILABLE: Naprelan, Permax, Zanaflex

COMPANY: Aventis Pharmaceuticals

PROGRAM ADDRESS: Aventis Oncology Pact Program
                        1101 King St. Suite 600
                        Alexandria VA 22314

TOLL FREE PHONE NUMBER: 800-996-6626

ELIGIBILITY: You cannot have insurance that provides prescription coverage and you must be ineligible for State Medicaid. Your income must be less than 250% (see pg. 249-250) of Federal Poverty Guidelines.

ENROLLMENT: Your doctor's office must calls to register you by phone, then a patient- and doctor-specific form is sent to your doctor.

FROM YOUR DOCTOR: Your doctor will complete the application, attach a prescription (if necessary), sign the application, and mail it to Aventis Pact Program.

WHAT YOU HAVE TO DO: Stay in contact with your doctor's office.

WHERE THE MEDICATION GOES: The medication will be sent to your doctor's office. The medication will not be sent to a P.O. Box.

AMOUNT GIVEN AT ONE TIME: Approval is usually within 48 hours. A 60-day supply, either 2 oral doses or an IV and an oral dose per chemo visit as specified under FDA approved use.

NO. OF REFILLS: Your doctor calls, completes, and faxes refill request for each additional 60-day supply. If your prescription has changed, a new order must be mailed in.

GENERAL INFORMATION: You can call between 9:00 am and 5:00 pm, Central Standard Time, Monday through Friday. This program is for labeled indication of the medication. If it is not being used for that, your doctor must request an exception through the manufacturer, this will take about a one (1) week longer.

MEDICATIONS AVAILABLE: Anzemet, Gliadel Wafers, Oncaspar, Taxotere

COMPANY: Axcan-Scandipharm, Inc.

PROGRAM ADDRESS: Axcan-Scandipharm, Inc.
                          22 Inverness Center Parkway
                          Birmingham, AL 35241

TOLL FREE PHONE NUMBER: 877-657-6737
ALTERNATIVE NUMBER: 800-742-6706

ELIGIBILITY: You cannot have insurance that provides prescription coverage and you must be ineligible for State Medicaid. You must have a diagnosis of Cystic Fibrosis, be between the ages of birth and 2 years of age.

ENROLLMENT: Your doctor's office should call for initial enrollment. The enrollment forms will be sent to your doctor.

FROM YOUR DOCTOR: Your doctor will complete the application, attach a prescription (if necessary), sign the application, and mail it to Axcan-Scandipharm.

WHAT YOU HAVE TO DO: Stay in contact with your doctor's office. Detailed financial and insurance information is required, including proof of your income and your total household income. Your signature is required.

WHERE THE MEDICATION GOES: The guardian will be given an ID number and a specific pharmacy to call. The medication will be mailed to your home. The medication will not be sent to a P.O. Box.

GENERAL INFORMATION: To receive ADEKs Pediatric Drops, ScandiShake, ScandiCal, you have to have purchased Ultrace. You can call between 9:00 am and 4:00 pm, Central Time, Monday through Friday.

MEDICATIONS AVAILABLE: ADEKs Pediatric Drops, ScandiShake, ScandiCal, Ultrace

COMPANY: Axcan-Scandipharm, Inc.

PROGRAM ADDRESS: Urso Patient Assistance Program
P.O. Box 52150
Phoenix, AZ 85072-2150

TOLL FREE PHONE NUMBER: 888-877-6471

ELIGIBILITY: You cannot have insurance that provides prescription coverage and you must be ineligible for State Medicaid. The program guidelines are based on Federal Poverty Guideline (see pg. 249-250), but they do not figure in prescription costs.

ENROLLMENT: Anyone may register you by phone. An Axcan case manager will take the information and do the initial screening. If you qualify (Axcan will not give out their exact guidelines), then the forms are mailed to you. Your household size, income, and prescription specifics will be needed when the call is made.

FROM YOUR DOCTOR: Your doctor will complete the application, attach a prescription (if necessary), sign the application, and mail it to Patient Assistance Program.

WHAT YOU HAVE TO DO: Stay in contact with your doctor's office. Detailed financial and insurance information is required, including proof of your income and your **total household** income. Your signature is required.

WHERE THE MEDICATION GOES: The medication will be sent from a mail order pharmacy directly to your home. The medication will not be sent to a P.O. Box.

AMOUNT GIVEN AT ONE TIME: Usually a 90-day supply.

NO. OF REFILLS: Your doctor can send in a prescription for up to a year. The product is shipped every 90 days. Additional forms are required after 6 months, a new application after one year.

GENERAL INFORMATION: You can call between 9:00 am and 5:00 pm, Eastern Time, Monday through Friday. The American Liver Foundation is underwriting a portion of this program.

MEDICATION AVAILABLE: Urso 250 mg

COMPANY: Axcan-Scandipharm, Inc.

PROGRAM ADDRESS: Viokase Patient Assistance Program
                      Attn. Customer Service
                      22 Inverness Center Parkway
                      Marietta, GA 30064

TOLL FREE PHONE NUMBER: 800-742-6706
ALTERNATIVE NUMBER: 800-472-2634 or 205-991-8085

ELIGIBILITY: You cannot have insurance that provides prescription coverage and you must be ineligible for State Medicaid.

ENROLLMENT: Your doctor's office should call for the form. Viokase Patient Assistance Program will fax the application to your doctor and copies of the form can be made.

FROM YOUR DOCTOR: Your doctor will complete the application, attach a prescription (if necessary), sign the application, and mail it to Viokase Patient Assistance Program. **The forms must be completed in blue ink.**

WHAT YOU HAVE TO DO: Stay in contact with your doctor's office. You must provide a copy of your prior year's tax return and copy of a denial letter from Medicaid or state assistance program The company will not make any exceptions regarding their requirements for copies of the tax returns and Medicaid denial letter. The other information needed for the form is minimal and would be on file with your doctor. You must sign the form.

WHERE THE MEDICATION GOES: The medication will be sent to your doctor's office. The medication will not be sent to a P.O. Box.

AMOUNT GIVEN AT ONE TIME: Usually a 120-day supply.

NO. OF REFILLS: Use a new form. There is a place on the back of the form to check off that the request is a refill.

GENERAL INFORMATION: You can call between 9:00 am and 4:00 pm, Eastern Time, Monday through Friday.

MEDICATIONS AVAILABLE: Viokase Powder, Viokase Tabs

COMPANY: Baxter Laboratories

PROGRAM ADDRESS: Baxter Patient Assistance Program
                            P.O. Box 1000
                            Building 200
                            Montville, NJ 07045

TOLL FREE PHONE NUMBER: 888-237-5394
FAX NUMBER: 973-305-3545

ELIGIBILITY: You cannot have insurance that provides prescription coverage and you must be ineligible for State Medicaid. Your adjusted gross must be below $20,000.00 per year. If you have insurance but no prescription coverage, your adjusted gross must be below $15,000.00 per year. You must be a U.S. citizen.

ENROLLMENT: Your doctor's office should call Baxter Laboratories. They will send or fax the application to your doctor.

FROM YOUR DOCTOR: Your doctor will complete the application, attach a prescription (if necessary), sign the application, and mail it to Baxter Laboratories.

WHAT YOU HAVE TO DO: Stay in contact with your doctor's office. You will have to provide financial and insurance information.

WHERE THE MEDICATION GOES: The medication will be sent to your doctor's office. The medication will not be sent to a P.O. Box.

AMOUNT GIVEN AT ONE TIME: Usually a 90-day supply.

GENERAL INFORMATION: You can call between 9:00 am and 4:00 pm, Eastern Time, Monday through Friday.

MEDICATIONS AVAILABLE: Feiba, Hemofil-M, Recombinate

COMPANY: Bayer Pharmaceutical

PROGRAM ADDRESS: Bayer Indigent Pharmaceutical Program
P.O. Box 29209
Phoenix, AZ 85028-9209

TOLL FREE PHONE NUMBER: 800-998-9180
FAX NUMBER: 602-808-7010

ELIGIBILITY: You cannot have insurance that provides prescription coverage and you must be ineligible for State Medicaid. You must be below the Federal Poverty Guideline (see pg. 249-250) levels to meet their guidelines. If there are extenuating circumstances, some time exceptions are made, so apply anyway.

ENROLLMENT: Your doctor's office should register you. This can be done by phone. Bayer will require your name, address, date of birth, social security number, number of individuals in your household, total household income and source, and fixed monthly medical expenses. Your doctor will provide the name of the medication, the dosage, and the strength.

If the need is immediate, your doctor is told to give you a prescription and have the pharmacist call the 1-800 number to get the benefit processing information and authorization to dispense the medication.

FROM YOUR DOCTOR: Your doctor will complete the application, attach a prescription (if necessary), sign the application, and mail it to Bayer Indigent Pharmaceutical Program.

WHAT YOU HAVE TO DO: Stay in contact with your doctor's office. You must go to your doctor's office to pick up the initial card, complete the card and sign your section of the form. Your must advise your doctor of any changes in your household income or insurance coverage.

WHERE THE MEDICATION GOES: By a pharmacy that participates in the RECAP Program.

AMOUNT GIVEN AT ONE TIME: Usually a 30-day supply.

GENERAL INFORMATION: You can call between 9:00 am and 4:00 pm, Mountain Time, Monday through Friday. When you are qualified, Bayer will send the form to your doctor. On lower left, of the form, there is a card your doctor and you must sign and date the form before it is taken to the pharmacy. Then take the temporary card to the pharmacy for a 30-day supply. After Bayer receives the form from the pharmacy, you will be sent a plastic card, which means an additional 60-day supply has been authorized. Then, Bayer will automatically authorize a 90-day supply every 90 days after that up to a year. There is no co-payment.

MEDICATIONS AVAILABLE: Adalat, Adalat CC, Ana Guard, ANA Kit, Biltricide, Chlo-Amine, Cipro, Cipro IV, Cipro Oral Suspension, Cort Dome Suppositories, Domepaste Bandages, DTIC Dome, Mezlin, Mithracin, MRV, Nimotope, Precose, Stilphostrol, Tridesilon Cream, Tridesilon Lotion, Venomil Maintenance

COMPANY: Beach Pharmaceuticals

PROGRAM ADDRESS: Beach Pharmaceuticals
                        5220 S. Manhattan Ave
                        Tampa, FL 33611

PHONE NUMBER: 813-839-6565

ELIGIBILITY: You cannot have insurance that provides prescription coverage and you must be ineligible for State Medicaid.

ENROLLMENT: Anyone can call for an enrollment application.

FROM YOUR DOCTOR: Your doctor will complete the application, attach a prescription (if necessary), sign the application, and mail it to Beach Pharmaceuticals.

WHAT YOU HAVE TO DO: Stay in contact with your doctor's office.

WHERE THE MEDICATION GOES: The medication will be sent to your doctor's office. The medication will not be sent to a P.O. Box.

AMOUNT GIVEN AT ONE TIME: Usually a 90-day supply.

GENERAL INFORMATION: You can call between 9:00 am and 4:00 pm, Eastern Time, Monday through Friday.

MEDICATIONS AVAILABLE: Beelith, Citrolith

COMPANY: Berlex Laboratories

PROGRAM ADDRESS: Berlex Patient Assistance Program
                            P.O. Box 1000
                            Building 200
                            Montville NJ 07045-1000

TOLL FREE PHONE NUMBER: 888-237-5394, #6
FAX NUMBER: 973-305-3545

ELIGIBILITY: You cannot have insurance that provides prescription coverage and you must be ineligible for State Medicaid. You must be a U.S. citizen with an adjusted gross income below $20,000, be ineligible for any public or private health insurance. If you have insurance but no prescription coverage then you must have an adjusted gross income less than $15,000.

ENROLLMENT: Your doctor's office must call for an enrollment application form.

FROM YOUR DOCTOR: Your doctor will complete both the physician's and patient portion of the enrollment application, attach a prescription (if necessary), sign the application, and mail it to Berlex Patient Assistance Program.

WHAT YOU HAVE TO DO: Stay in contact with your doctor's office. You will need to provide detailed income and insurance information.

WHERE THE MEDICATION GOES: The medication will be sent to your doctor's office. The medication will not be sent to a P.O. Box.

AMOUNT GIVEN AT ONE TIME: Usually a 90-day supply.

GENERAL INFORMATION: Betapace AF is shipped in bottles of 60. You can call between 9:00 am and 4:00 pm, Eastern Time, Monday through Friday.

MEDICATIONS AVAILABLE: Betapace 80 mg, Betapace 120 mg, Betapace 160 mg, Betapace 240 mg, Climara, Quinaglute–Dura Tabs 324 mg.

COMPANY: Berlex Laboratories

PROGRAM ADDRESS: Fludara Patient Assistance Program
1101 King St.
Suite 600
Alexandria, Va. 22314

TOLL FREE PHONE NUMBER: 888-237-5394

ELIGIBILITY: You cannot have insurance that provides prescription coverage. With an adjusted salary of $27,000.00 per year for a single person and an adjusted, gross salary of $40,000.00 with dependents.

ENROLLMENT: Your doctor's office will have to call and register you for the program. They will send the application forms to your doctor.

FROM YOUR DOCTOR: Your doctor will complete the application, attach a prescription (if necessary), sign the application, and mail it to Fludara Patient Assistance Program.

WHAT YOU HAVE TO DO: Stay in contact with your doctor's office. You will have to provide financial and non-coverage information.

WHERE THE MEDICATION GOES: The medication will be sent to your doctor's office. The medication will not be sent to a P.O. Box.

AMOUNT GIVEN AT ONE TIME: Up to 5 vials per month for 6 months.

GENERAL INFORMATION: You can call between 9:00 am 4:00 pm, Eastern Time, Monday through Friday.

MEDICATION AVAILABLE: Fludara

COMPANY: Bertek Pharmaceuticals, Inc.

PROGRAM ADDRESS: Bertek Pharmaceuticals, Inc.
                        781 Chestnut Ridge Rd.
                        Morgantown, WV 26505

TOLL FREE PHONE NUMBER: 888-823-7835, ext 4043

ELIGIBILITY: You cannot have insurance that provides prescription coverage and you must be ineligible for State Medicaid. Your household income for a family of 1 (one) must be under $8,740. A family household income for 2 (two) must be under $11,060. A family household income for 3 (three) must be under $13,860. A family household income for 4 (four) must be under $16,700.

ENROLLMENT: Anyone may call to enroll you. The forms will be sent to your doctor.

FROM YOUR DOCTOR: Your doctor will complete the application, attach a prescription (if necessary), sign the application, and mail it to Bertek Pharmaceuticals, Inc.

WHAT YOU HAVE TO DO: Stay in contact with your doctor's office. You must sign the forms. You will be required to provide financial information.

WHERE THE MEDICATION GOES: The medication will be sent to your doctor's office. The medication will not be sent to a P.O. Box.

AMOUNT GIVEN AT ONE TIME: Usually a 90-day supply. Maxzide, Maxzide-25, and Clorpes are filled with stock bottles of 100's. Nitrek is filled with stock packages of 30.

GENERAL INFORMATION: You must be U.S. residents. You can call between 9:00 am and 4:00 pm, Eastern Time, Monday through Friday.

MEDICATIONS AVAILABLE: Clorpes, Maxzide, Maxzide-25, Nitrek

COMPANY: Biogen

PROGRAM ADDRESS: Nova Factor, Inc.
                                   1620 Century Center Parkway, Suite 109
                                   Memphis TN 38134

TOLL FREE PHONE NUMBER: 800-456-2255

ELIGIBILITY: You must have remitting/relapsing Multiple Sclerosis (MS). Your adjusted gross annual household income must be below $72,000.00 per year. If you have no insurance or insurance without prescription coverage, you will have to pay a $25 shipping fee every 3 months. If you have only Medicare, you pay $895.00 for 1 year with no shipping costs, which can be paid in monthly payments. They offer a sliding scale for patients who can't afford their co-insurance fees. Depending on your income and insurance status, cost sharing may be required. This can be done by either purchasing your share of the medication from a local pharmacy or by utilizing the Avonex Direct Delivery Program. You must be a U.S. resident.

ENROLLMENT: Anyone can call and talk to a reimbursement specialist about the Access Program and enroll you in the program.

FROM YOUR DOCTOR: Your doctor will complete the application, along with a signed statement of medical necessity, and mail it to Nova Factor, Inc. The application serves as prescription. If necessary, your doctor will arrange injection training for you or for who will be giving you the injection.

WHAT YOU HAVE TO DO: Stay in contact with your doctor's office. You will have to provide detailed financial and insurance information. You will have to sign the enrollment application.

WHERE THE MEDICATION GOES: The drug will be sent directly to your home. The medication will not be sent to a P.O. Box.

AMOUNT GIVEN AT ONE TIME: A 90-day supply, 3 packets of 4 weekly injections. This will be refilled four (4) times.

GENERAL INFORMATION: You can call between 8:30 am and 5:00 pm, Central Time, Monday through Friday.

MEDICATION AVAILABLE: Avonex

COMPANY: Blaine Company, Inc.

PROGRAM ADDRESS: Blaine Company, Inc.
                            1515 Production Drive
                            Burlington, KY 41005

TOLL FREE PHONE NUMBER: 800-633-9353
ALTERNATIVE NUMBER: 606-283-9437
FAX NUMBER: 606-283-9460

ELIGIBILITY: You cannot have insurance that provides prescription coverage and you must be ineligible for State Medicaid. You must be under the prescribing care of a cardiologist, internist or a transplant clinic. No co-payment is required.

ENROLLMENT: A nurse, social worker, or your doctor can contact the program and ask for an application. The application will be mailed or faxed **only** to your doctor. It can be copied.

FROM YOUR DOCTOR: Your doctor will complete the application, attach a prescription (if necessary), sign the application, and mail it Blaine Company, Inc.

WHAT YOU HAVE TO DO: Stay in contact with your doctor's office.

WHERE THE MEDICATION GOES: The medication will be sent to your doctor's office. The medication will not be sent to a P.O. Box.

AMOUNT GIVEN AT ONE TIME: One bottle of 120 pills, or 10 strips of 10 pills

TIME TO GET MEDICATION: It will take up to three weeks.

NO. OF REFILLS: Use an entirely new application, just like the first time.

GENERAL INFORMATION: You can call between 9:00 am and 4:00 pm, Central Time, Monday through Friday.

MEDICATIONS AVAILABLE: Mag-Ox 400 mg, Uro-Mag 140 mg Capsules

COMPANY: Boehringer Ingelheim

PROGRAM ADDRESS: Boehringer Ingelheim Partners in Health
                      Program 900 Ridgebury Rd.
                      P.O. Box 368
                      Ridgefield, CT 06877-0368

TOLL FREE PHONE NUMBER: 800-556-8317
ALTERNATIVE NUMBER: 203-798-4131

ELIGIBILITY: You cannot have insurance that provides prescription coverage and you must be ineligible for State Medicaid. You must be a U.S. citizen and a U.S. resident. The income guidelines for this program are very low. The income limits are: $750 per month for one person ($9,000/yr.); $1,000 per month for 2 people ($12,000/yr.); $1,250 per month for 3 people ($15,000/yr.); and $1,500 per month for 4 people ($18,000/yr).

ENROLLMENT: Anyone can call for the enrollment application. The forms will be sent to your doctor.

FROM YOUR DOCTOR: Your doctor will complete the application, attach a prescription (if necessary), sign the application, and mail it to Boehringer Ingelheim Partners in Health.

WHAT YOU HAVE TO DO: Stay in contact with your doctor's office. You will have to provide detailed financial and insurance information.

WHERE THE MEDICATION GOES: The medication will be sent to your doctor's office. The medication will not be sent to a P.O. Box.

AMOUNT GIVEN AT ONE TIME: Usually a 90-day supply.

TIME TO GET MEDICATION: 2-3 weeks

GENERAL INFORMATION: A physician can only have **THREE** patients enrolled in program at one time and only one product per patient. You can call between 9:00 am and 4:00 pm, Eastern Time, Monday through Friday.

MEDICATIONS AVAILABLE: Aggrenox, Alupent Inhalation Aerosol, Alupent Inhalation Solution, Alupent Tabs, Alupent Syrup, Atrovent Inhalation Aerosol, Atrovent Inhalation Solution, Atrovent Nasal Spray 0.03%, Atrovent Nasal Spray 0.06%, Catapres-TTS patch (NOT Catapres pills), Combivent Inhalation Aerosol, Flomax, Mexitil, Micardis, Mobic, Serentil Tabs (for FDA approved uses)

COMPANY: Bristol-Myers-Squibb

PROGRAM ADDRESS: Access Program
                                       6900 College Blvd.
                                       Suite 1000
                                       Overland Park, KS 66211-9840

TOLL FREE PHONE NUMBER: 800-437-0994
FAX NUMBER: 888-776-2370

ELIGIBILITY: You cannot have insurance that provides prescription coverage and you must be ineligible for State Medicaid.

ENROLLMENT: Anyone can call for an enrollment application. The Access Program will send the forms to your doctor.

FROM YOUR DOCTOR: Your doctor will complete the application, attach a prescription (if necessary), sign the application, and mail it to the Access Program.

WHAT YOU HAVE TO DO: Stay in contact with your doctor's office. You will have to provide detailed financial and insurance information. You must sign the application.

WHERE THE MEDICATION GOES: The medication will be sent to your doctor's office. The medication will not be sent to a P.O. Box.

AMOUNT GIVEN AT ONE TIME: Usually a 90-day supply.

NO. OF REFILLS: The application is good for 6 months.

GENERAL INFORMATION: You can call between 8:30 am and 5:00 pm, Central Time, Monday through Friday. Your doctor can request up to 3 products on one application. The application is patient- and doctor-specific.

MEDICATIONS AVAILABLE: BiCNU, Blenoxane, CeeNU, Cytoxan Tablets, Cytoxan Lyophilized IV, Fungizone, Hydrea, Iflex/Mesna, Lysodren, Megace Tablets, Megace Oral Suspension, Mesnex, Mutamycin, Mycostatin Oral Suspension, Mycostatin Tabs, Paraplatin, Platinol-AQ, Rubex, Taxol, Teslac, VePesid, Videx Pediatric Oral Powder, Videx Oral Suspension, Vumon, Zerit, Zerit Oral

COMPANY: Bristol-Myers-Squibb

PROGRAM ADDRESS: Patient Assistance Foundation
                     c/o HDS
                     P.O. Box 52001
                     Phoenix, AZ 85072-9160

TOLL FREE PHONE NUMBER: 800-736-0003
FAX NUMBER: 800-344-8792

ELIGIBILITY: You cannot have insurance that provides prescription coverage and you must be ineligible for State Medicaid. Your income must be below 200% of the Federal Poverty Guideline (see pg. 249-250).

ENROLLMENT: Anyone can call for an enrollment application. The application will be sent to your doctor.

FROM YOUR DOCTOR: Your doctor will complete the application, attach a prescription (if necessary), sign the application, and mail it to Patient Assistance Foundation.

WHAT YOU HAVE TO DO: Stay in contact with your doctor's office. You will have to provide detailed financial and insurance information. You must sign the application.

WHERE THE MEDICATION GOES: The medication will be sent to your doctor's office. The medication will not be sent to a P.O. Box.

AMOUNT GIVEN AT ONE TIME: Usually a 90-day supply.

GENERAL INFORMATION: You can call between 9:00 am and 6:00 pm, Eastern Time, Monday through Friday.

MEDICATIONS AVAILABLE: Avalide, Avapro, BuSpar, BuSpar Dividose, Capoten, Capozide, Cefzil Oral Suspension, Cefzil Tabs, Cogard, Corzide 40/5 Tabs, Corzide 80/5 Tabs, Delestrogen, Deseryl, Duricef, Dynapen, Estrace Vaginal Cream, Florinef, Glucophage, Kantrex, Kenalog Capsules, Kenalog Tabs, Kenalog Aerosol Spray, Kenalog Cream, Kenalog Lotion, Kenalog Ointment, Kenalog Pediatric Injection, Kenalog-10, Kenalog-40, Kenalog-in-Orabase, Klotrix, K-Lyte DS, K-Lyte CL, Monopril, Monopril-HCT, Mucomyst, Mucomyst-10, Mucomyst-20, Mycolog II Cream, Mycolog II Lotion, Mycostatin, Naldecon Ligui-Gel, Naldecon Pediatric Drops, Naldecon Pediatric Syrup, Naldecon Syrup, Naldecon Tabs, Naturetin, Nydrazid, Plavix, Pravachol, Prolixin Decanoate Injectable, Prolixin Oral, Pronestyl Capsules, Pronestyl Suspension, Pronestyl Tabs, Pronestyl-SR, Questran Oral, Questran Light, Questran Suspension, Rauzide, Serzone, Tequin, Theragran Hematinic, Ultravate, Vasodilan

COMPANY: BTG Pharmaceuticals

PROGRAM ADDRESS: BTG Pharmaceuticals
                        Patient Assistance Program
                        P.O. Box 221887
                        Charlotte, NC 28222-1887

TELEPHONE NUMBER: 876-692-6374

ELIGIBILITY: You cannot have insurance that provides prescription coverage and you must be ineligible for State Medicaid. You must be a resident of the U.S.

ENROLLMENT: Anyone can call for an enrollment application form.

FROM YOUR DOCTOR: Your doctor will complete the application, attach a prescription for a 30-day supply (with two (2) refills), sign the application, and mail it to BTG Pharmaceuticals.

WHAT YOU HAVE TO DO: Stay in contact with your doctor's office.

WHERE THE MEDICATION GOES: The medication will be sent to your doctor's office. The medication will not be sent to a P.O. Box.

AMOUNT GIVEN AT ONE TIME: Usually a 90-day supply.

GENERAL INFORMATION: There are income guidelines. You can call between 9:00 am and 4:00 pm, Eastern Time, Monday through Friday.

MEDICATION AVAILABLE: Oxandrin

COMPANY: Carnrick Laboratories

PROGRAM ADDRESS: Carnrick Laboratories
                       65 Horse Hill Rd.
                       Cedar Knolls, NJ 07927

ALTERNATIVE NUMBER: 973-267-2670

ELIGIBILITY: You cannot have insurance that provides prescription coverage and you must be ineligible for State Medicaid. Your income must be under the Federal Poverty Guideline (see pg. 249-250).

ENROLLMENT: Anyone can call and enroll you in the program. The application will be sent to your doctor.

FROM YOUR DOCTOR: Your doctor will complete the application, attach a prescription (if necessary), sign the application, and mail it to Carnrick Laboratories.

WHAT YOU HAVE TO DO: Stay in contact with your doctor's office. You will have to provide detailed financial and insurance information. You will have to sign the application.

WHERE THE MEDICATION GOES: The medication will be sent to your doctor's office. The medication will not be sent to a P.O. Box.

AMOUNT GIVEN AT ONE TIME: Usually a 90-day supply, but it depends on the medication.

GENERAL INFORMATION: You can call between 9:00 am and 4:00 pm, Eastern Time, Monday through Friday.

MEDICATIONS AVAILABLE: Amen, Bontril PDM, Bontril SR, Exgest LA, Hydrocet, Midrin, Motofen, Nolahist, Nolamine Time Release, Phrenilin Forte, Propagest, Salflex, Sinulin, Skelaxin, Theo-X ER

COMPANY: Carter Wallace Laboratories

PROGRAM ADDRESS: Carter Wallace Laboratories
                         P.O. Box 1001
                         Cranbury, NJ 08512

ALTERNATIVE NUMBER: 609-655-6000

ELIGIBILITY: You cannot have insurance that provides prescription coverage and you must be ineligible for State Medicaid.

ENROLLMENT: Your doctor's office has to call and enroll you in the program. The application will be sent to your doctor.

FROM YOUR DOCTOR: Your doctor will complete the application, attach a prescription (if necessary), sign the application, and mail it to Carter Wallace Laboratories. Your doctor must not be charging you for services.

WHAT YOU HAVE TO DO: Stay in contact with your doctor's office. You will have to provide detailed financial and insurance information. You will have to sign the application.

WHERE THE MEDICATION GOES: The medication will be sent to your doctor's office. The medication will not be sent to a P.O. Box.

AMOUNT GIVEN AT ONE TIME: Usually a 90-day supply.

GENERAL INFORMATION: Patients with Medicare will not qualify for the program. You can call between 9:00 am and 4:00 pm, Eastern Time, Monday through Friday.

MEDICATION AVAILABLE: Felbatol

COMPANY: Celgene Corporation

PROGRAM ADDRESS: Celgene Corporation
                            Thalomid Patient Assistance Program
                            7 Powder Horn Drive
                            Warren, NJ 07059

TOLL FREE PHONE NUMBER: 888-423-5436

ELIGIBILITY: You cannot have insurance that provides prescription coverage and you must be ineligible for State Medicaid.

ENROLLMENT: Anyone can call and enroll you in the program. They will need detailed financial and insurance information at the time of enrollment. The application will be sent to your doctor.

FROM YOUR DOCTOR: Your doctor will complete the application, attach a prescription (if necessary), sign the application, and mail it to Celgene Thalomid Patient Assistance Program.

WHAT YOU HAVE TO DO: Stay in contact with your doctor's office. You will have to provide detailed financial and insurance information. You will have to sign the application.

WHERE THE MEDICATION GOES: The medication will be sent to your doctor's office. The medication will not be sent to a P.O. Box.

AMOUNT GIVEN AT ONE TIME: A 28-day cycle.

NO. OF REFILLS: After 6 months, Celgene Thalomid Patient Assistance Program will contact you and re-interviews you to re-establish eligibility.

GENERAL INFORMATION: You can call between 9:00 am and 4:00 pm, Eastern Time, Monday through Friday.

MEDICATION AVAILABLE: Thalomid

COMPANY: Centocor, Inc.

PROGRAM ADDRESS: Centocor, Inc.
                           Remicade Patient Assistance Program
                           4733 Main Street
                           Suite 201
                           Lisle, IL 60532

TOLL FREE PHONE NUMBER: 800-964-8345
FAX NUMBER: 800-281-7384

ELIGIBILITY: You cannot have insurance that provides prescription coverage and you must be ineligible for State Medicaid.

ENROLLMENT: Your doctor's office must call for an enrollment application form. The enrollment application will only be faxed to your doctor's office.

FROM YOUR DOCTOR: Your doctor will complete the application, attach a prescription (if necessary), sign the application, and fax it to Remicade Patient Assistance Program.

WHAT YOU HAVE TO DO: Stay in contact with your doctor's office. You will have to provide financial and insurance information.

WHERE THE MEDICATION GOES: The medication will be sent to your doctor's office. The medication will not be sent to a P.O. Box.

AMOUNT GIVEN AT ONE TIME: It will depend on the diagnosis, usually a 90-day supply.

GENERAL INFORMATION: You can re-apply every six months. You can call between 9:00 am and 4:00 pm, Central Time, Monday through Friday.

MEDICATION AVAILABLE: Remicade

COMPANY: Centocor, Inc.

PROGRAM ADDRESS: Centocor Solutions for Retavase
                               1800 Robert Fulton Drive
                               Suite 300
                               Reston, VA 20191

TOLL FREE PHONE NUMBER: 800-331-5773

ELIGIBILITY: You cannot have insurance that provides prescription coverage and you must be ineligible for State Medicaid.

ENROLLMENT: Centocor prefers a hospital professional to call and enroll you. The person calling should have the patient's chart available.

FROM YOUR DOCTOR: An authorized hospital personnel completes, signs the form, and mails it to Centocor Solutions for Retavase.

WHAT YOU HAVE TO DO: You will have to provide detailed financial and insurance information. You will have to sign the application.

WHERE THE MEDICATION GOES: This program provides replacement product to the hospital.

GENERAL INFORMATION: This drug is for the treatment of acute heart attacks and is an injectable medicine. The program has two components: One is wastage and breakage replacement. The product has to be mixed prior to use and once mixed can't be reused. In instances where the drug was mixed and then not used or if the vial was broken, the company will provide a replacement vial. The other part of the program is patient assistance—it's a reimbursement-type program.

GENERAL INFORMATION: You can call between 9:00 am and 4:00 pm, Eastern Time, Monday through Friday.

MEDICATION AVAILABLE: Retavase

COMPANY: Cephalon, Inc.

PROGRAM ADDRESS: Provigil Assistance Program
                        145 Brandywine Parkway
                        West Chester, PA 19380-4245

TOLL FREE PHONE NUMBER: 800-675-8415
ALTERNATIVE NUMBER: 610-344-0200
FAX NUMBER: 610-344-0063

ELIGIBILITY: You cannot have insurance that provides prescription coverage and you must be ineligible for State Medicaid. You must have a diagnosis of Narcolepsy.

ENROLLMENT: Anyone can call and enroll you in the program. The application will be sent to your doctor.

FROM YOUR DOCTOR: Your doctor will complete the application, attach a prescription (if necessary), sign the application, and mail it to Provigil Assistance Program.

WHAT YOU HAVE TO DO: Stay in contact with your doctor's office. You will have to provide detailed financial and insurance information. You will have to sign the application.

WHERE THE MEDICATION GOES: The medication will be sent to your doctor's office. The medication will not be sent to a P.O. Box.

AMOUNT GIVEN AT ONE TIME: Usually a 90-day supply.

GENERAL INFORMATION: There is a 50% co-payment. You can call between 9:00 am and 4:00 pm, Eastern Time, Monday through Friday.

MEDICATION AVAILABLE: Provigil

COMPANY: Cetylite Industries, Inc.

PROGRAM ADDRESS: Cetylite Industries, Inc.
P.O. Box 90006
Pennsauken, NJ 08110

TOLL FREE PHONE NUMBER: 800-257-7740
ALTERNATIVE NUMBER: 609-665-6111
FAX NUMBER: 609-665-5408

ELIGIBILITY: You cannot have insurance that provides prescription coverage and you must be ineligible for State Medicaid.

ENROLLMENT: Anyone may can to enroll you.

FROM YOUR DOCTOR: Your doctor will complete the application, attach a prescription (if necessary), sign the application, and mail it to Cetylite Industries, Inc.

WHAT YOU HAVE TO DO: Stay in contact with your doctor's office.

WHERE THE MEDICATION GOES: The medication will be sent to your doctor's office. The medication will not be sent to a P.O. Box.

GENERAL INFORMATION: Very limited information. You can call between 9:00 am and 4:00 pm, Eastern Time, Monday through Friday.

MEDICATION AVAILABLE: Cetacaine Topical

COMPANY: Chiron Therapeutics

PROGRAM ADDRESS: Chiron Reimbursement Service
                            c/o The Lewin Group
                            490 Second St, Suite 201
                            San Francisco, CA 94107

TOLL FREE PHONE NUMBER: 800-775-7533
ALTERNATIVE NUMBER: 800-244-7668

ELIGIBILITY: You cannot have insurance that provides prescription coverage and you must be ineligible for State Medicaid. You must be a U.S. citizen or a legal U.S. resident to be eligible.

ENROLLMENT: Your doctor's office must call the program prior to the patient beginning therapy. Initial eligibility screening is done over the phone and then a patient-specific form is faxed to the prescribing physician. For RabAvert, the drug is ordered immediately after screening and the application and attachments must be returned before the patient completes the RabAvert treatment.

FROM YOUR DOCTOR: Your doctor will complete the application, attach a prescription (if necessary), sign the application, and mail it to Chiron Reimbursement Service. If the form is **not properly and completely** filled out, it will be returned, delaying the process.

WHAT YOU HAVE TO DO: Stay in contact with your doctor's office. You must provide detailed financial and insurance information. You must sign the form.

WHERE THE MEDICATION GOES: The medication will be sent to your doctor's office. The medication will not be sent to a P.O. Box.

GENERAL INFORMATION: You can call between 9:00 am and 4:00 pm, Pacific Time, Monday through Friday.

MEDICATIONS AVAILABLE: DepoCyt, Proleukin, RabAvert

COMPANY: COR Therapeutics

PROGRAM ADDRESS: COR Therapeutics
256 East Grand Ave.
South San Francisco, CA 94080

TOLL FREE PHONE NUMBER: 888-267-4533
ALTERNATIVE NUMBER: 650-244-6812

ELIGIBILITY: You cannot have insurance that provides prescription coverage and you must be ineligible for State Medicaid.

ENROLLMENT: The doctor or the institution contacts the local COR Therapeutics representative for an enrollment form.

FROM YOUR DOCTOR: Your doctor will complete the application, attach a prescription (if necessary), sign the application, and mail it to COR Therapeutics.

WHAT YOU HAVE TO DO: Stay in contact with your doctor's office.

WHERE THE MEDICATION GOES: The medication will be sent to your doctor's office. The medication will not be sent to a P.O. Box.

GENERAL INFORMATION: You must meet the FDA product indication guidelines. This program provides reimbursement product. COR Therapeutics' preference is that the provider requests multiple copies of the form from the representative rather than make copies. You can call between 9:00 am and 4:00 pm, Pacific Time, Monday through Friday.

MEDICATION AVAILABLE: Intergilin injectable

COMPANY: Dermik Laboratories

PROGRAM ADDRESS: Dermik Laboratories
                        500 Arcola Rd
                        P.O. Box 1200
                        Collegeville, PA 19426-0107

TOLL FREE PHONE NUMBER: 800-727-6737
ALTERNATIVE NUMBER: 702-353-4100

ELIGIBILITY: You cannot have insurance that provides prescription coverage and you must be ineligible for State Medicaid.

ENROLLMENT: Your doctor's office will call the company and request an enrollment form.

FROM YOUR DOCTOR: Your doctor will complete the application, attach a prescription (if necessary), sign the application, and mail it to Dermik Laboratories.

WHAT YOU HAVE TO DO: Stay in contact with your doctor's office. You will have to provide detailed income and insurance information. You must sign the application.

WHERE THE MEDICATION GOES: The medication will be sent to your doctor's office. The medication will not be sent to a P.O. Box.

AMOUNT GIVEN AT ONE TIME: Usually a 90-day supply.

GENERAL INFORMATION: Their income guidelines are somewhat above the poverty level but would not be specific. You can call between 9:00 am and 4:00 pm, Eastern Time, Monday through Friday.

MEDICATIONS AVAILABLE: Benzagel 10 Acne Gel, Benzagel 5 Acne Gel, Benzamycin Gel, Drithocreme 0.10% HP Cream, Drithocreme 0.25% HP Cream, Drithocreme 0.50% HP Cream, Drithocreme 1.0% HP Cream, Dritho-Scalp, Florone, Florone E, Hytone Cream, Hytone Lotion, Hytone Ointment, Klaron Lotion, Penlac, Psorcon .05% Cream, Psorcon .05% Ointment, Psorcon Cream E, Psorcon Ointment E, Sulfacet-R Lotion, Vanoxide-HC Lotion, Vytone Cream, Zetar Emulsion

COMPANY: Dista Products

PROGRAM ADDRESS: Lilly Cares
P.O. Box 25768
Alexandria, VA 22313

TOLL FREE PHONE NUMBER: 800-545-6962 (For forms)
ALTERNATIVE NUMBER: 800-545-5979 (For customer
service)

ELIGIBILITY: You cannot have insurance that provides prescription coverage and you must be ineligible for State Medicaid.

ENROLLMENT: Anyone may call for an enrollment application, but it is sent only to the doctor.

FROM YOUR DOCTOR: Your doctor will complete the application, attach a prescription (if necessary), sign the application, and mail it to Lilly Cares.

WHAT YOU HAVE TO DO: Stay in contact with your doctor's office. You must provide income and insurance information and sign the form.

WHERE THE MEDICATION GOES: The medication will be sent to your doctor's office. The medication will not be sent to a P.O. Box. For some medication, certificates or vouchers are sent and you take them to the pharmacy.

AMOUNT GIVEN AT ONE TIME: Usually a 90-day supply.

GENERAL INFORMATION: You can call between 9:00 am and 4:00 pm, Eastern Time, Monday through Friday.

MEDICATIONS AVAILABLE: Ilosone, Ilotycin, Ilotycin Ophthalmic Ointment, Keflex Oral Suspension, Keflex Pulvules, Keftab, Prozac Liquid, Prozac Oral, Prozac Pulvules

COMPANY: Dupont Pharma Company

PROGRAM ADDRESS: Dupont Pharma Company
                         Chestnut Run Plaza, Hickory Run Bldg.
                         974 Center Rd.
                         Wilmington, DE 19880-0723

TOLL FREE PHONE NUMBER: 800-474-2762
ALTERNATIVE NUMBER: 302-992-4240
                         800-390-1735 (For Lotensin)

ELIGIBILITY: You cannot have insurance that provides prescription coverage and you must be ineligible for State Medicaid.

ENROLLMENT: Anyone can call for the enrollment application form.

FROM YOUR DOCTOR: Your doctor will complete the application, attach a prescription (if necessary), sign the application, and mail it to Dupont Pharma Company.

WHAT YOU HAVE TO DO: Stay in contact with your doctor's office. You will have to provide income and insurance information. You must sign the application.

WHERE THE MEDICATION GOES: The medication will be sent to your doctor's office. The medication will not be sent to a P.O. Box.

AMOUNT GIVEN AT ONE TIME: A 6-month supply in quantities of 100s for Coumadin and Simement, a 3-month supply for Revia in quantities of 30 pills.

GENERAL INFORMATION: You can call between 9:00 am and 5:00 pm, Eastern Time, Monday through Friday. Lotensin is not yet commercially available but your doctor can receive free samples.

MEDICATIONS AVAILABLE: Coumadin, Lodosyn, Lotensin, Revia, Simement, Simement CR

COMPANY: Dupont-Merck

PROGRAM ADDRESS: Dupont-Merck
Patient Assistance Program
P.O. Box 222157
Charlotte, NC 28222

TOLL FREE PHONE NUMBER: 800-334-4486 Ext. 216
ALTERNATIVE NUMBER: 800-474-2762
FAX NUMBER: 888-441-9012

ELIGIBILITY: You cannot have insurance that provides prescription coverage and you must be ineligible for State Medicaid.

ENROLLMENT: Anyone can call for an enrollment application form. The application form will be sent to your doctor's office.

FROM YOUR DOCTOR: Your doctor will complete the enrollment application, attach three (3) one (1) month prescriptions, sign the application, and mail it to Dupont-Merck.

WHAT YOU HAVE TO DO: Stay in contact with your doctor's office.

WHERE THE MEDICATION GOES: The medication will be sent to your doctor's office. The medication will not be sent to a P.O. Box.

AMOUNT GIVEN AT ONE TIME: A 30-day supply.

NO. OF REFILLS: 4

GENERAL INFORMATION: You can call between 9:00 am-6:00 pm, Eastern Time, Monday through Friday.

MEDICATION AVAILABLE: Sustiva

COMPANY: Dura Pharmaceuticals, Inc.

PROGRAM ADDRESS: Dura Pharmaceuticals, Inc.
                              7474 Lusk Blvd
                              San Diego, CA 92121

TOLL FREE PHONE NUMBER   888-859-8583
ALTERNATE PHONE NUMBER   619-457-2553
FAX NUMBER: 619-457-3211

ELIGIBILITY: You cannot have insurance that provides prescription coverage and you must be ineligible for State Medicaid.

ENROLLMENT: Your doctor's office needs to call the company for the enrollment process.

FROM YOUR DOCTOR: Your doctor will complete the application, attach a prescription (if necessary), sign the application, and mail it to Dura Pharmaceuticals, Inc.

WHAT YOU HAVE TO DO: Stay in contact with your doctor's office. You must sign the form.

WHERE THE MEDICATION GOES: The medication will be sent to your doctor's office. The medication will not be sent to a P.O. Box.

AMOUNT GIVEN AT ONE TIME: Usually a 90-day supply.

GENERAL INFORMATION: You can call between 8:00 am and 5:00 pm, Pacific Time, Monday through Friday.

MEDICATION AVAILABLE: Myanbutol

COMPANY: ECR Pharmaceuticals

PROGRAM ADDRESS: ECR Pharmaceuticals
P.O. Box 71600
Richmond, VA 23255

TOLL FREE PHONE NUMBER: 800-527-1955
ALTERNATIVE NUMBER: 804-527-1950
FAX NUMBER: 804-527-1959

ELIGIBILITY: You cannot have insurance that provides prescription coverage and you must be ineligible for State Medicaid.

ENROLLMENT: Your doctor's office contacts the area representative.

FROM YOUR DOCTOR: Your doctor must write a letter on office letterhead stating your needs and lack of prescription coverage. Your doctor must attach a prescription to the letter before mailing it to ECR Pharmaceuticals. If there is an ECR Pharmaceuticals representative in the area, your doctor may just explain the situation to him/her.

WHAT YOU HAVE TO DO: Stay in contact with your doctor's office.

WHERE THE MEDICATION GOES: The medication will be sent to your doctor's office. The medication will not be sent to a P.O. Box.

AMOUNT GIVEN AT ONE TIME: Usually a 90-day supply.

GENERAL INFORMATION: You can call between 9:00 am and 4:00 pm, Eastern Time, Monday thru Friday.

MEDICATIONS AVAILABLE: Anaplex 30 mg, Anaplex 60 mg, Anaplex DM Cough Syrup, Anaplex HD Cough Syrup, Anaplex SR, Bupap, Deepak, Lodrane Allergy Capsules, Lodrane LD Capsules, Lodrane Liquid, Nasatab LA Tablets, Panalgesic Gold Cream, Panalgesic Gold Liniment, Pneumotussin HC Cough Syrup, Pneumotussin Tablets, Taper Pak

COMPANY: Elan Pharmaceuticals, Inc.

PROGRAM ADDRESS: Athena Rx Home Pharmacy
                           800 Gateway Boulevard
                           S. San Francisco, CA 94080

TOLL FREE PHONE NUMBER: 800-537-8899

ELIGIBILITY: You cannot have insurance that provides prescription coverage and you must be ineligible for State Medicaid. You must be a resident of the U.S. Your net worth must be less than $30,000.

ENROLLMENT: Your doctor's office must call for an enrollment application form.

FROM YOUR DOCTOR: Your doctor must write a letter on office stationery stating your need for the medication, your financial situation, the medication will be used according to FDA labeling requirements, attach a prescription and mail it to Athena Rx Home Pharmacy.

WHAT YOU HAVE TO DO: Stay in contact with your doctor's office. You will have to provide detailed income and insurance information.

WHERE THE MEDICATION GOES: The medication will be sent to your doctor's office. The medication will not be sent to a P.O. Box.

AMOUNT GIVEN AT ONE TIME: Usually a 90-day supply.

GENERAL INFORMATION: You can call between 9:00 am and 4:00 pm, Pacific Time, Monday through Friday.

MEDICATIONS AVAILABLE: Diastat, Mysoline Suspension, Mysoline Tabs, Naprelan, Permax, Zanaflex, Zonegran

COMPANY: Eli Lilly and Company

PROGRAM ADDRESS: Lilly Cares Program Administrator
                       P.O. Box 25768
                       Alexandria, VA 22313

TOLL FREE PHONE NUMBER: 800-545-6962
ALTERNATIVE NUMBER: 800-545-5979

ELIGIBILITY: You cannot have insurance that provides prescription coverage and you must be ineligible for State Medicaid.

ENROLLMENT: They will only send the applications directly to your doctor's office. Your doctor should call for the application.

FROM YOUR DOCTOR: Your doctor will complete the application, attach a prescription (if necessary), sign the application, and mail it to Lilly Cares Program Administrator.

WHAT YOU HAVE TO DO: Stay in contact with your doctor's office. You will have to provide your exact income and source. DO NOT STATE ZERO INCOME. Be as specific as you can to your situation. **Otherwise, the form will be sent back!**

WHERE THE MEDICATION GOES: The medication will be sent to your doctor's office. The medication will not be sent to a P.O. Box.

AMOUNT GIVEN AT ONE TIME: Insulin users receive a voucher good for 3 months' supply at their pharmacy with $2.00 co-pay each month.

GENERAL INFORMATION: You can call between 9:00 am and 4:00 pm, Eastern Time, Monday through Friday.

MEDICATIONS AVAILABLE: Atropine Sulfate, Aventyl HCL Liquid, Aventyl HCL Pulvules, Calcium Carbonate, Ceclor Pulvules, Ceclor Suspension, Dobutrex Solution, Evista, Gemzar, Glucagon, Humalog, Humatrope, Humulin (all types), Iletin II Lente, Iletin II NPH, Ilosone, Ilotycocin, Keflex, Keftab, Kefurox, Lorabid Pulvules, Lorabid Suspension, Mandol Vials, Oncovin Solution, Protamine Sulfate, Prozac, Quinidine Gluconate, Reo Pro Vials, Sodium Bicarbonate Tablets, Tubocurarine Chloride Vials, Vancocin HCL Oral, Vancocin HCL Pulvules, Velban

COMPANY: Eli Lilly and Company

PROGRAM ADDRESS: Reliance Prescription Support Program
          P.O. Box 6842
          Somerset, NJ 08875

TOLL FREE PHONE NUMBER: 800-792-2737

ELIGIBILITY: You cannot have insurance that provides prescription coverage and you must be ineligible for State Medicaid.

ENROLLMENT: Anyone can call for an enrollment application form but the form will only be sent to your doctor's office.

FROM YOUR DOCTOR: Your doctor will complete the enrollment application, attach a prescription (if necessary), sign the application, and mail it to Reliance Prescription Support Program.

WHAT YOU HAVE TO DO: Stay in contact with your doctor's office. You will have to provide detailed financial and insurance information. You must sign the application.

WHERE THE MEDICATION GOES: The medication will be sent to your doctor's office. The medication will not be sent to a P.O. Box.

AMOUNT GIVEN AT ONE TIME: Usually a 90-day supply.

TIME TO GET MEDICATION: About three (3) weeks.

NO. OF REFILLS: 4

GENERAL INFORMATION: You can call between 9:00 am and 4:00 pm, Eastern Time, Monday through Friday. This is a temporary program and a program of last resort. Eligibility is determined by a formula. Your application should include a letter of denial from Medicaid or your insurance company. This will save you time since they will require a letter of denial at some point in the application process.

MEDICATIONS AVAILABLE: Axid, Dynacire

COMPANY: Eli Lilly and Company

PROGRAM ADDRESS: Lilly Cares Program Administrator
                            Eli Lilly & Co.-Zyprexa Program
                            P.O. Box 25768
                            Alexandria, VA 22313

TOLL FREE PHONE NUMBER: 800-488-2133
ALTERNATIVE NUMBER: 800-545-6962, 800-545-5979
FAX NUMBER: 703-317-5618

ELIGIBILITY: You cannot have insurance that provides prescription coverage and you must be ineligible for State Medicaid.

ENROLLMENT: Anyone can call to enroll you but they will need your name, address, phone number, social security number, number of people in the household, source and dollar amount of your income, dollar amount of monthly out-of-pocket expenses and dollar amount of liquid assets, insurance status, and disability status. The form will only be sent to a physician.

FROM YOUR DOCTOR: Your doctor will complete the application, attach a prescription (if necessary), sign the application, and mail it to Lilly Cares Program Administrator.

WHAT YOU HAVE TO DO: Stay in contact with your doctor's office. You must sign the application.

WHERE THE MEDICATION GOES: The medication will be sent to your doctor's office. The medication will not be sent to a P.O. Box.

AMOUNT GIVEN AT ONE TIME: Usually a 90-day supply.

GENERAL INFORMATION: You can call between 8:30 am and 5:00 pm, Eastern Time, Monday through Friday.

MEDICATION AVAILABLE: Zyprexa

COMPANY: ESI Lederle, Inc.

PROGRAM ADDRESS: ESI Lederle, Inc.
Wyeth-Ayerst Labs
P.O. Box 41502
Philadelphia, PA 19101

TOLL FREE PHONE NUMBER: 800-395-9938
ALTERNATIVE NUMBER: 800-934-5556

ELIGIBILITY: You cannot have insurance that provides prescription coverage and you must be ineligible for State Medicaid.

ENROLLMENT: Anyone can call for an application.

FROM YOUR DOCTOR: Your doctor will complete the application, attach a prescription (if necessary), sign the application, and mail it to ESI Lederle, Inc.

WHAT YOU HAVE TO DO: Stay in contact with your doctor's office. You must sign the form.

WHERE THE MEDICATION GOES: The medication will be sent to your doctor's office. The medication will not be sent to a P.O. Box.

AMOUNT GIVEN AT ONE TIME: A 90-day supply.

GENERAL INFORMATION: You can call between 9:00 am and 4:00 pm, Eastern Time, Monday through Friday.

MEDICATIONS AVAILABLE: Aygestin, Cycrin

COMPANY: Faulding Laboratories

PROGRAM ADDRESS: Faulding Laboratories
                         Patient Assistance Program
                         5511 Capital Dr.
                         Suite 550
                         Raleigh, NC 27606

TOLL FREE PHONE NUMBER: 919-233-5375

ELIGIBILITY: You cannot have insurance that provides prescription coverage and you must be ineligible for State Medicaid.

ENROLLMENT: Anyone can call for an enrollment application form. The form will be sent to your doctor's office.

FROM YOUR DOCTOR: Your doctor will complete the enrollment application, attach a prescription (if necessary), sign the application, and mail it to Faulding Laboratories.

WHAT YOU HAVE TO DO: Stay in contact with your doctor's office. You will have to provide detailed financial information.

WHERE THE MEDICATION GOES: The medication will be sent to your doctor's office. The medication will not be sent to a P.O. Box.

AMOUNT GIVEN AT ONE TIME: Usually a 90-day supply.

NO. OF REFILLS: Up to a year before having to reapply.

GENERAL INFORMATION: You can call between 9:00 am and 4:00 pm, Eastern Time, Monday through Friday.

MEDICATION AVAILABLE: Kadian C-11

COMPANY: Ferndale Laboratories, Inc.

PROGRAM ADDRESS: Ferndale Laboratories, Inc.
                              780 West Eight Mile Rd.
                              Ferndale, MI 48220

TOLL FREE PHONE NUMBER: 800-621-6003 ext 707
ALTERNATIVE NUMBER: 248-548-0900
FAX NUMBER: 248-548-0708

ELIGIBILITY: You cannot have insurance that provides prescription coverage and you must be ineligible for State Medicaid.

ENROLLMENT: They have no formal program but have been known to help. Your doctor's office should call to explain your circumstances.

FROM YOUR DOCTOR: Your doctor will complete the application, attach a prescription (if necessary), sign the application, and mail it to Ferndale Laboratories, Inc.

WHAT YOU HAVE TO DO: Stay in contact with your doctor's office.

WHERE THE MEDICATION GOES: The medication will be sent to your doctor's office. The medication will not be sent to a P.O. Box.

GENERAL INFORMATION: You can call between 9:00 am and 4:00 pm, Eastern Time, Monday through Friday.

MEDICATIONS AVAILABLE: Analpram Rectal Cream 1%, Analpram Rectal Cream 2.5%, Analpram Lotion, Kronofed-A Kronocaps, Kronofed-A Jr. Kronocaps, Locoid Cream, Locoid Ointment, Locoid Topical Lotion, Locoid Lipocream C Cream, Promosone Cream, Promosone Ointment, Promosone Topical Lotion

COMPANY: Ferring Pharmaceuticals, Inc.

PROGRAM ADDRESS: Ferring Pharmaceuticals, Inc.
                         Customer Services
                         120 White Plains Rd., Suite 400
                         Tarrytown, NY 10591

TOLL FREE PHONE NUMBER: 888-337-7464
ALTERNATIVE NUMBER: 888-793-6367

ELIGIBILITY: You cannot have insurance that provides prescription coverage and you must be ineligible for State Medicaid.

ENROLLMENT: Your doctor's office must call and talk with the reimbursement specialist.

FROM YOUR DOCTOR: Your doctor will complete the application, attach a prescription (if necessary), sign the application, and mail it to Ferring Pharmaceuticals, Inc. The doctor must demonstrate that you must have the drug for quality of life and you cannot afford the medication.

WHAT YOU HAVE TO DO: Stay in contact with your doctor's office.

WHERE THE MEDICATION GOES: The medication will be sent to your doctor's office. The medication will not be sent to a P.O. Box.

GENERAL INFORMATION: Coverage depends on the your state guidelines. If Medicaid doesn't cover the drug needed, then the company will try to get the state to cover its cost or they will try to find another reimbursement source. If an insurance program covers you, the company will determine why the drug isn't paid for. Providing the drug at no cost is a last resort because none of their medications are used to treat life-threatening illnesses and most of their drugs are indictable that should be covered by insurance. You can call between 9:00 am and 4:00 pm, Eastern Time, Monday through Friday.

MEDICATIONS AVAILABLE: Acthrel, Desmopressin Acetate Injection, Desmopressin Acetate Rhinal Tube, Lutrepulse, Repronex, Secretin-Ferring, Thyrel TRH

COMPANY: Forest Pharmaceuticals, Inc.

PROGRAM ADDRESS: Forest Pharmaceuticals, Inc.
                                     Indigent Care Program
                                     13600 Shoreline Drive
                                     St. Louis, MO 63045

TOLL FREE PHONE NUMBER: 800-851-0758
FAX NUMBER: 314-493-7452

ELIGIBILITY: You cannot have insurance that provides prescription coverage and you must be ineligible for State Medicaid.

ENROLLMENT: Anyone can call for an enrollment application form.

FROM YOUR DOCTOR: Your doctor will complete the application (including DEA number), a diagnosis, attach a prescription (if necessary), sign the application, and mail it to Forest Pharmaceuticals, Inc.

WHAT YOU HAVE TO DO: Stay in contact with your doctor's office. You will have to provide detailed financial and insurance information. You must sign the enrollment application.

WHERE THE MEDICATION GOES: The medication will be sent to your doctor's office. The medication will not be sent to a P.O. Box.

AMOUNT GIVEN AT ONE TIME: Usually a 90-day supply.

GENERAL INFORMATION: Total household income is required. You can call between 9:00 am and 4:00 pm, Central Time, Monday through Friday.

MEDICATIONS AVAILABLE: Aerobid Inhaler System, Aerobid-M Inhaler System, AeroChamber, AeroChamber with Mask, Armour Thyroid, Celexa, Esgic Capsules, Esgic Tabs, Esgic Plus, Kay Ciel Oral Suspension, Kay Ciel Powder Packets, Levothroid, Nitrogard, Tessalon Perls, Theochron, Thyrolar, Tiazac

COMPANY: Fujisawa USA, Inc.

PROGRAM ADDRESS: Fujisawa USA, Inc.
                         3 Parkway North Center
                         Deerfield, IL 60015-2548

TOLL FREE PHONE NUMBER: 800-727-7003

ELIGIBILITY: You cannot have insurance that provides prescription coverage and you must be ineligible for State Medicaid.

ENROLLMENT: Your doctor's office needs to start the enrollment process.

FROM YOUR DOCTOR: Your doctor needs to writes a letter on office stationery, stating your need and your lack of prescription coverage. A prescription is required. Mail it to Fujisawa USA, Inc.

WHAT YOU HAVE TO DO: Stay in contact with your doctor's office. You will need to give your doctor your financial and insurance information. This information must accompany the letter from the doctor.

WHERE THE MEDICATION GOES: The medication will be sent to your doctor's office. The medication will not be sent to a P.O. Box.

AMOUNT GIVEN AT ONE TIME: Usually a 90-day supply.

GENERAL INFORMATION: You can call between 9:00 am and 4:00 pm, Central Time, Monday through Friday.

MEDICATIONS AVAILABLE: Adenoscan, Aristocort Cream A .025%, Aristocort Cream A .01%, Aristocort Cream A .50%, Aristocort Ointment A .1%, Aristocort Suspension, Cefizox, Cyclocort, Elase Ointment, Elase-Chloromycetin Ointment, Promosone Ointment, Promosone Suspension

COMPANY: Fujisawa USA, Inc.

PROGRAM ADDRESS: Fujisawa USA
                             Prograf Patient Assistant Program
                             c/o Intelecenter
                             P.O. Box 4133
                             Gaithersburg, MD 20878-5355

TOLL FREE PHONE NUMBER: 800-477-4723
ALTERNATIVE NUMBER: 800-477-6472,
                                        202-393-5563

ELIGIBILITY: You cannot have insurance that provides prescription coverage and you must be ineligible for State Medicaid.

ENROLLMENT: Your doctor's office must call for an enrollment application form.

FROM YOUR DOCTOR: Your doctor will complete the application, attach a prescription (if necessary), sign the application, and mail it to Prograf Patient Assistant Program.

WHAT YOU HAVE TO DO: Stay in contact with your doctor's office. You must provide income and insurance information.

WHERE THE MEDICATION GOES: The medicine is sent from a program-affiliated mail-order pharmacy. The medication will not be sent to a P.O. Box.

AMOUNT GIVEN AT ONE TIME: Two (2) 90-day shipments. You will be billed $20 per shipment.

GENERAL INFORMATION: Households with incomes of less than $35,000 are eligible as long as they have no prescription coverage. The company is the payer of last resort. You can call between 9:00 am and 4:00 pm, Eastern Time, Monday through Friday.

MEDICATION AVAILABLE: Prograf

COMPANY: Galderma Laboratories

PROGRAM ADDRESS: Galderma Laboratories
                         Patient Assistance Program
                         14501 N. Freeway
                         Ft. Worth, TX 76177

TOLL FREE PHONE NUMBER: 800-582-8225

ELIGIBILITY: You cannot have insurance that provides prescription coverage and you must be ineligible for State Medicaid.

ENROLLMENT: Your doctor's office needs to start the enrollment process.

FROM YOUR DOCTOR: Your doctor will write a letter on letterhead stationery stating your need, lack of prescription coverage, attach a prescription, and mail it to Galderma Laboratories.

WHAT YOU HAVE TO DO: Stay in contact with your doctor's office.

WHERE THE MEDICATION GOES: The medication will be sent to your doctor's office. The medication will not be sent to a P.O. Box.

AMOUNT GIVEN AT ONE TIME: Usually a 90-day supply.

GENERAL INFORMATION: You can call between 9:00 am and 4:00 pm, Central Time, Monday through Friday.

MEDICATIONS AVAILABLE: MetroCream, MetroGel, MetroLotion

COMPANY: Gates Pharmaceutical

PROGRAM ADDRESS: Gates Pharmaceutical
650 Cathill Rd
Sellersville, PA 18960

TOLL FREE PHONE NUMBER: 800-292-4283
FAX NUMBER: 215-653-0839

ELIGIBILITY: You cannot have insurance that provides prescription coverage and you must be ineligible for State Medicaid.

ENROLLMENT: Anyone can call for an enrollment application form.

FROM YOUR DOCTOR: Your doctor will complete the application, attach a prescription (if necessary), sign the application, and mail it to Gates Pharmaceutical.

WHAT YOU HAVE TO DO: Stay in contact with your doctor's office. You will have to provide proof of income.

WHERE THE MEDICATION GOES: The medication will be sent to your doctor's office. The medication will not be sent to a P.O. Box.

AMOUNT GIVEN AT ONE TIME: Usually a 90-day supply.

GENERAL INFORMATION: You can call between 9:00 am and 4:00 pm, Eastern Time, Monday through Friday.

MEDICATIONS AVAILABLE: Galzin, Orap

COMPANY: Genentech, Inc.

PROGRAM ADDRESS: Genentech, Inc.
                         Uninsured Patient Assistance Program
                         P.O. Box 2586, Mail Stop #13
                         South San Francisco, CA 94083-2586

TOLL FREE PHONE NUMBER: 800-530-3083
ALTERNATIVE NUMBER: 415-225-1000
FAX NUMBER: 415-225-1366

ELIGIBILITY: You cannot have insurance that provides prescription coverage and you must be ineligible for State Medicaid. For Activase, the patient's income must be less than $30,000.

ENROLLMENT: For Activase ONLY: The hospital must apply for reimbursement product, **one-time basis.** For all other products, your doctor must call for an enrollment application form.

FROM YOUR DOCTOR: Your doctor will complete the application, attach a prescription (if necessary), sign the application, and mail it to Genentech, Inc.

WHAT YOU HAVE TO DO: Stay in contact with your doctor's office.

WHERE THE MEDICATION GOES: The medication will be sent to your doctor's office. The medication will not be sent to a P.O. Box.

AMOUNT GIVEN AT ONE TIME: Usually a 90-day supply.

GENERAL INFORMATION: For Activase, the application is completed by the hospital and the product is supplied to reimburse the hospital for treating the patient. The date of service must be within one year of the application. You can call between 8:00 am and 5:00 pm, Pacific Time, Monday through Friday.

MEDICATIONS AVAILABLE: Activase, Herceptin, Nutropin, Nutropin AQ, Protropin, Rituxan

COMPANY: Genentech, Inc.

PROGRAM ADDRESS: Genentech Endowment for Cystic Fibrosis
                        4828 Parkway Plaza Blvd.
                        Suite 120
                        Charlotte, NC 28217-1969

TOLL FREE PHONE NUMBER: 800-297-5557

ELIGIBILITY: You must have Cystic Fibrosis. Genentech, Inc., has three (3) separate programs: There is a program for people with no insurance, individuals who are unable to pay the insurance co-payments, or for individuals who have insurance available to them but cannot afford the coverage. Each program has its own set pre-established criteria based on financial situation, insurance coverage and medical necessity.

ENROLLMENT: Anyone can call for an enrollment application form.

FROM YOUR DOCTOR: Your doctor will complete the application, attach a prescription (if necessary), sign the application, and mail it to Genentech Endowment for Cystic Fibrosis.

WHAT YOU HAVE TO DO: Stay in contact with your doctor's office. You must complete and sign the enrollment application.

WHERE THE MEDICATION GOES: You will receive a voucher to use with a mail order pharmacy. The medication shipped to directly to you.

AMOUNT GIVEN AT ONE TIME: A 30-day supply.

GENERAL INFORMATION: You can call between 8:00 am and 5:00 pm, Eastern Time, Monday through Friday. These programs may provide full or partial assistance. They will also provide assistance to purchase the nebulizer and compressors used in Pulmozyme administration

MEDICATION AVAILABLE: Pulmozyme

COMPANY: Geneva Pharmaceuticals

PROGRAM ADDRESS: Geneva Pharmaceuticals
Patient Support Program
556 Morris Ave.
D-2058
Summit, NJ 07091

TOLL FREE PHONE NUMBER: 800-257-3273

ELIGIBILITY: You cannot have insurance that provides prescription coverage and you must be ineligible for State Medicaid. You must be a U.S. resident.

ENROLLMENT: Anyone can call for an enrollment application form. The enrollment application will be sent to your doctor.

FROM YOUR DOCTOR: Your doctor will complete the application, attach a prescription (if necessary), sign the application, and mail it to Geneva Pharmaceuticals.

WHAT YOU HAVE TO DO: Stay in contact with your doctor's office. You may be asked to provide financial and insurance information. You must sign the enrollment application.

WHERE THE MEDICATION GOES: The medication will be sent to your doctor's office. The medication will not be sent to a P.O. Box.

AMOUNT GIVEN AT ONE TIME: Usually a 90-day supply.

GENERAL INFORMATION: You can call between 9:00 am and 4:00 pm, Eastern Time, Monday through Friday.

MEDICATIONS AVAILABLE: Actigall, Anafranil, Anturane, Apresazide, Apresoline, Aredia, Brethaire Inhaler, Brethine, Cataflam, Cytadren, Desferal, Esidrix, Esimil, Estraderm, Habitrol, Ismelin, Lamprene, Lioresal, Lopressor, Lopressor HCT, Lotensin, Lotensin HCT, Lotrel, Ludiomil, PBZ, PBZ-ER Tabs, Regitine, Rimactene, Ser-Ap-Es, Slow-K, Tegretol Chewable Tabs, Tegretol PM Capsules, Tegretol Suspension, Tegretol Tabs, Tegretol XR Tabs, Tofranil, Tofranil-PM, Transderm-SCOP, Transdermal-Nitro, Voltaren Tabs, Voltaren XR Tabs

COMPANY: Genzyme Therapeutics

PROGRAM ADDRESS: Medical Affairs
Genzyme Corp.
One Kendall Square
Cambridge, MA 0213

TOLL FREE PHONE NUMBER: 800-745-4447, x7808
FAX NUMBER: 617-252-7700

ELIGIBILITY: You cannot have insurance that provides prescription coverage and you must be ineligible for State Medicaid.

ENROLLMENT: Your doctor **(PERSONALLY, not an office representative)** must call for an enrollment application form.

FROM YOUR DOCTOR: Your doctor will complete the application, attach a prescription (if necessary), sign the application, and mail it to Genzyme Corp.

WHAT YOU HAVE TO DO: Stay in contact with your doctor's office. You will have to provide detailed financial and insurance information.

WHERE THE MEDICATION GOES: The medication will be sent to your doctor's office. The medication will not be sent to a P.O. Box.

AMOUNT GIVEN AT ONE TIME: Usually a 90-day supply.

GENERAL INFORMATION: The Company has case managers who help patients by providing assistance with reimbursement and will look for other organizations or charities to cover the cost. If all else fails, the company has a compassionate use program. Medicare should cover Cerezyme. You can call between 9:00 am and 4:00 pm, Eastern Time, Monday through Friday.

MEDICATIONS AVAILABLE: Cerezyme, Renagel

COMPANY: Gilead Sciences Corporation

PROGRAM ADDRESS: Gilead Sciences Support Services
                            333 Lakeside Drive
                            Foster City, CA 94404

TOLL FREE PHONE NUMBER: 800-226-2056
ALTERNATIVE NUMBER: 800-445-3235, option 6
FAX NUMBER: 800-216-6857

ELIGIBILITY: You cannot have insurance that provides prescription coverage and you must be ineligible for State Medicaid.

ENROLLMENT: Anyone can call for an enrollment application form. The form will be sent directly to your doctor.

FROM YOUR DOCTOR: Your doctor will complete the application, attach a prescription (if necessary), sign the application, and mail it to Gilead Sciences Support Services.

WHAT YOU HAVE TO DO: Stay in contact with your doctor's office. Your signature is required.

WHERE THE MEDICATION GOES: The medication will be sent to your doctor's office. The medication will not be sent to a P.O. Box.

AMOUNT GIVEN AT ONE TIME: Usually a 90-day supply.

GENERAL INFORMATION: You can call between 9:00 am and 5:30 pm, Eastern Time, Monday through Friday. They will provide insurance claims assistance and advocacy for patients. They will also help physicians in getting authorization from third party payers, will provide advocacy for the patient to the insurance companies, and assist with appeals. **They do not provide direct assistance.**

MEDICATIONS AVAILABLE: DaunoXome, Vistide

COMPANY: Glaxo Wellcome, Inc.

PROGRAM ADDRESS: Glaxo Wellcome, Inc.
                      Patient Assistance Program
                      P.O. Box 52185
                      Phoenix, AZ 85072-9711

TOLL FREE PHONE NUMBER: 800-722-9294
ALTERNATIVE NUMBER: 800-745-2967
FAX NUMBER: 800-750-9832

ELIGIBILITY: You cannot have insurance that provides prescription coverage and you must be ineligible for State Medicaid.

ENROLLMENT: Anyone can call for an enrollment application form. They will send a form to your doctor but the form can't be copied

FROM YOUR DOCTOR: Your doctor will complete the application, attach a prescription (if necessary), sign the application, and mail it to Glaxo Wellcome, Inc.

WHAT YOU HAVE TO DO: Stay in contact with your doctor's office. You will have to provide financial information and sign the form.

WHERE THE MEDICATION GOES: You will receive a card to take your pharmacy and receive the medication.

AMOUNT GIVEN AT ONE TIME: Once eligibility is determined, the tear-off card on the application is good for a 30-day supply.

GENERAL INFORMATION: You can call between 9:00 am and 9:00 pm, Eastern Time, Monday through Friday or between 9:00 am and 5:30 pm, on Saturday. Some products have a $5 co-pay, some have a $10 co-pay. Glaxo-Wellcome also provides advocacy for insurance reimbursement.

MEDICATIONS AVAILABLE: Aclovate Cream, Aclovate Lotion, Agenerase Capsules, Agenerase Oral, Alkeran, Amerge, Baclofen, Beclovent Inhalation Aerosol, Beconase Inhalation System, Beconase AQ Nasal Spray, Ceftin, Ceptaz, Combivir, Cutivate Cream, Cutivate Ointment, Daraprim, Epivir Tabs, Epivir-HBV Oral Suspension, Epivir-HBV Tabs, Epivir Optic Solution, Flolan, Flonase Nasal Spray, Flovent Nasal Spray, Flovent 44 mcg Inhalation Aerosol, Flovent 110 mcg Inhalation Aerosol, Flovent 220 mcg Inhalation Aerosol, Flovent Rotadisk 50 mcg, Flovent Rotadisk 100 mcg, Flovent Rotadisk 250 mcg, Fortaz, Imitrex Injectable, Imitrex Nasal Spray, Imitrex Tabs, Lamictal Tabs, Lamictal Chewable Tabs, Lanoxicaps, Lanoxin, Lanoxin Elixir (Pediatric), Lanoxin Injectable, Lanoxin Injectable (Pediatric), Leukeran Oral, Lotronex, Mepron, Myleran, Navelbine, Nuromax, Oxistat Cream, Oxistat Lotion, Purinethol, Retrovir Capsules, Retrovir Tabs, Retrovir Syrup, Serevent Inhalation Aerosol, Serevent Diskus, Temovate Cream, Temovate Lotion, Temovate Ointment, Temovate E Emollient, Temovate Scalp Application, Thioguanine, Valtrex, Vasoxyl, Ventolin, Wellbutrin, Wellbutrin SR, Zantac 150 Tabs, Zantac 150 Capsules, Zantac 150 EFFERdose Granules, Zantac 150 EFFERdose Tabs, Zantac 150 Geldose Capsules, Zantac 300 Geldose Capsules, Zantac Syrup, Zantac Injectable, Zantac Premix Injectable, Ziagen Oral Solution, Ziagen Tabs, Zinacef Tabs, Zinacef Oral Solution, Zinacef Injectable, Zinacef Premix Injectable, Zofran SR, Zovirax SR, Zyban

COMPANY: Hoechst Marion Roussel, Inc.

PROGRAM ADDRESS: Hoechst Marion Roussel, Inc.
Indigent Patient Program
P.O. Box 9627
Kansas City, MO 64134-0950

TOLL FREE PHONE NUMBER: 800-221-4025
ALTERNATIVE NUMBER: 800-552-3656

ELIGIBILITY: You cannot have insurance that provides prescription coverage and you must be ineligible for State Medicaid. Your household income levels must be below: one (1) member, less than $8,050 per year ($670 per month), two (2) members, less than $10,850 per year ($904 per month), for each additional family member add $2,800 per year ($233 per month).

ENROLLMENT: Anyone can call for an enrollment application form. The enrollment application form will only be faxed to your doctor.

FROM YOUR DOCTOR: Your doctor will complete the application, attach a prescription (if necessary), sign the application, and mail it to Hoechst Marion Roussel, Inc. Hoechst Marion Roussel, Inc., encourages doctors to waive their fees.

WHAT YOU HAVE TO DO: Stay in contact with your doctor's office. You will have to provide detailed financial information including income and insurance, if any.

WHERE THE MEDICATION GOES: The medication will be sent to your doctor's office. The medication will not be sent to a P.O. Box. Your name will be on the shipping label.

AMOUNT GIVEN AT ONE TIME: Usually a 90-day supply.

GENERAL INFORMATION: Rifadin, Rifamate, Rifater are not available for the treatment of TB. You can call between 9:00 am and 4:00 pm, Central Time, Monday through Friday.

MEDICATIONS AVAILABLE: Allegra, Allegra D, Amaryl, Arava, Bentyl Capsules, Bentyl Syrup, Bentyl Tabs, Cantil, Carafate Capsules, Carafate Suspension, Carafate Tabs, Cardizem, Cardizem CD, Cardizem SR, Cephulac 10 gm, Cephulac 15 ml, Chronulac Lactulose Syrup, Claforan, Clomid, DiaBeta, Hiprex, Lasix, Norpramin, Novafed A, Rifadin, Rifamate, Rifater, Trental

COMPANY:　　　　　　Hoechst Marion Roussel, Inc.

PROGRAM ADDRESS:　　Anzemet Indigent Patient
　　　　　　　　　　　　Assistance Program
　　　　　　　　　　　　CRC, Inc.
　　　　　　　　　　　　8990 Springbrook Drive, Suite 200
　　　　　　　　　　　　Minneapolis, MN 55433

TOLL FREE PHONE NUMBER:　888-895-2219

ELIGIBILITY: You cannot have insurance that provides prescription coverage and you must be ineligible for State Medicaid. Your household income level must be less than $20,125 for a household of one ($1,677 per month), $27,125 for a household of two or more ($2,260 per month).

ENROLLMENT: Anyone can call for an enrollment application form. Your doctor will have to call to register you. The form is patient- and doctor-specific.

FROM YOUR DOCTOR: Your doctor will complete the application, attach a prescription (if necessary), sign the application, and mail it to Anzemet Indigent Patient Assistance Program.

WHAT YOU HAVE TO DO: Stay in contact with your doctor's office. You will have to provide income and insurance information.

WHERE THE MEDICATION GOES: The medication will be sent to your doctor's office. The medication will not be sent to a P.O. Box.

AMOUNT GIVEN AT ONE TIME: Usually a 90-day supply.

GENERAL INFORMATION: You can call between 9:00 am and 4:00 pm, Central Time, Monday through Friday.

MEDICATION AVAILABLE: Anzemet

COMPANY: Hoechst Marion Roussel, Inc.

PROGRAM ADDRESS: Hoechst Marion Roussel, Inc.
                           Nilandron Patient Assistance Program
                           P.O. Box 9627
                           Kansas City, MO 64134-9950

TOLL FREE PHONE NUMBER: 800-221-4025 #3
ALTERNATIVE NUMBER: 800-522-3656

ELIGIBILITY: You cannot have insurance that provides prescription coverage and you must be ineligible for State Medicaid. Their income guidelines are: For a one (1) person household, income must fall below $8050 per year ($670 per month); for a two (2) person household, income must fall below $10,850 per year ($901) per month), **OR** you are experiencing special circumstances.

ENROLLMENT: Anyone can call for an enrollment application form. They will fax the enrollment application only to your doctor.

FROM YOUR DOCTOR: Your doctor will complete the application, attach a prescription (if necessary), sign the application, and mail it to Nilandron Patient Assistance Program.

WHAT YOU HAVE TO DO: Stay in contact with your doctor's office. You will have to provide detailed financial information or explain the special circumstances.

WHERE THE MEDICATION GOES: The medication will be sent to your doctor's office. The medication will not be sent to a P.O. Box.

AMOUNT GIVEN AT ONE TIME: Usually a 90-day supply.

GENERAL INFORMATION: There are very strict financial guidelines and most people are not going to qualify for assistance "experiencing special circumstances," a good catch phrase for denial. You can call between 9:00 am and 4:00 pm, Central Time, Monday through Friday.

MEDICATION AVAILABLE: Nilandron

COMPANY: Horizon Pharmaceuticals

PROGRAM ADDRESS: Horizon Pharmaceuticals
                          660 Henbree Parkway
                          Suite 106
                          Roswell, GA 30076

TOLL FREE PHONE NUMBER: 800-849-9707 ext. 321
ALTERNATIVE NUMBER: 770-442-9707

ELIGIBILITY: You cannot have insurance that provides prescription coverage and you must be ineligible for State Medicaid. You must be a resident of the U.S. Your income has to be at or below Federal Poverty Guideline (see pg. 249-250).

ENROLLMENT: Your doctor's office must call for an enrollment application form. The application will be sent to your doctor's office.

FROM YOUR DOCTOR: Your doctor will complete the enrollment application, attach a prescription (if necessary), sign the application, and mail it to First Horizon Pharmaceuticals.

WHAT YOU HAVE TO DO: Stay in contact with your doctor's office. You will have to provide detailed financial information.

WHERE THE MEDICATION GOES: The medication will be sent to your doctor's office. The medication will not be sent to a P.O. Box.

AMOUNT GIVEN AT ONE TIME: Nitrolingual: 1 pump with 200 pre-measured doses per year. Robinul: 100 tablets per year. Cognex: A 90-day supply at a time.

GENERAL INFORMATION: You can call between 9:00 am and 4:00 pm, Eastern Time, Monday through Friday. You will have a $7.00 co-pay. This co-pay must accompany the original application and will be refunded if you are denied assistance.

MEDICATIONS AVAILABLE: Cognex, Nitrolingual Pumpspray, Robinul, Robinul Forte

COMPANY: ICN Pharmaceuticals, Inc.

PROGRAM ADDRESS: ICN Pharmaceuticals, Inc.
                        ICN Plaza
                        3300 Hyland Ave.
                        Costa Mesa, CA 92626

TOLL FREE PHONE NUMBER: 800-556-1937, option 4
ALTERNATIVE NUMBER: 714-545-0100
FAX NUMBER;   714-641-7289

ELIGIBILITY: You cannot have insurance that provides prescription coverage and you must be ineligible for State Medicaid.

ENROLLMENT: Anyone can call for an enrollment application form. The enrollment application form will only be sent to your doctor.

FROM YOUR DOCTOR: Your doctor will complete the application, attach a prescription (if necessary), sign the application, and mail it to ICN Pharmaceuticals, Inc.

WHAT YOU HAVE TO DO: Stay in contact with your doctor's office.

WHERE THE MEDICATION GOES: The medication will be sent to your doctor's office. The medication will not be sent to a P.O. Box.

AMOUNT GIVEN AT ONE TIME: Usually a 90-day supply.

GENERAL INFORMATION: You can call between 8:00 am and 5:00 pm, Pacific Time, Monday through Friday. They will only provide a three (3) months' supply of medication per year. Unless your doctor writes a letter indicating you will need more than a three (3) months' supply.

MEDICATIONS AVAILABLE: 8-MOP Capsules, Ancobon, Benoquin Cream, Efudex Cream, Efudex Topical Solution, Eldopaque Forte Cream, Eldoquin Forte Cream, Fototar Cream, Oxsoralen Lotion, Oxsoralen-Ultra Capsules, Solaquin Forte Cream, Solaquin Forte Gel, Tensilon Injectable, Virazole, Vitadye Lotion

COMPANY: ICN Pharmaceuticals, Inc.

PROGRAM ADDRESS: Myasthenia Gravis Association
of Western Pennsylvania
1323 Forbes Ave.,
Suite 201
Pittsburgh, PA 15219

TOLL FREE PHONE NUMBER: 800-783-7615

ELIGIBILITY: You cannot have insurance that provides prescription coverage and you must be ineligible for State Medicaid. You will need a letter of denial from Medicaid. They will authorize a 90-day supply if they know that the denial letter is pending and know that the patient is going to be denied.

ENROLLMENT: Anyone can call for an enrollment application form. They would prefer you use an original enrollment application because they are color coded according to medication.

FROM YOUR DOCTOR: Your doctor will complete the application, attach a prescription (if necessary), sign the application, and mail it to Myasthenia Gravis Association of Western Pennsylvania. Your doctor must sign and return the "receipt of goods" form once the medication is received. This is in order for you to be eligible for another shipment

WHAT YOU HAVE TO DO: Stay in contact with your doctor's office. You will have to provide detailed income and insurance information. The denial letter from Medicaid is required. You must sign the enrollment application.

WHERE THE MEDICATION GOES: The medicine is sent either to the doctor's office or to a pharmacy that has agreed not to charge a dispensing fee. The medication will not be sent to a P.O. Box.

AMOUNT GIVEN AT ONE TIME: Usually a 90-day supply.

GENERAL INFORMATION: This association runs the patient assistance program for ICN Pharmaceuticals, Inc. You do not have to live in Western Pennsylvania. You can call between 9:00 am and 4:00 pm, Eastern Time, Monday through Friday.

MEDICATIONS AVAILABLE: Mestinon Injectable, Mestinon Syrup, Mestinon Tablets, Mestinon Timespan Tablets, Prostigmin Injectable

COMPANY: Immunex Corporation

PROGRAM ADDRESS: Immunex Corporation
51 University St.
Seattle, WA 98101

TOLL FREE PHONE NUMBER: 800-321-4669
FAX NUMBER: 800-944-3184

ELIGIBILITY: You cannot have insurance that provides prescription coverage and you must be ineligible for State Medicaid. You must be a U.S. citizen or legal U.S. resident (including U.S. territories). You must be below stated income levels: household of one (1): $24,720 per year ($2,068 per month). For a household of two (2): $33,180 per year ($2,765 per month).

ENROLLMENT: Your doctor's office must contact Immunex Corporation before you begin therapy. They will not enroll patients retroactively. They will do an initial screening and fax your doctor a patient-specific enrollment application packet that cannot be copied.

FROM YOUR DOCTOR: Your doctor will complete the application, attach a prescription (if necessary), sign the application, and the area representative must also sign the form, and mail or fax it to Immunex Corporation. The Hotline will notify the physician regarding eligibility within 24 hours of receipt. **(Incomplete applications will be returned, causing a delay.)**

WHAT YOU HAVE TO DO: Stay in contact with your doctor's office. You will have to provide detailed income and insurance information. You must sign the enrollment application.

WHERE THE MEDICATION GOES: The medication will be sent to your doctor's office. The medication will not be sent to a P.O. Box.

AMOUNT GIVEN AT ONE TIME: Usually a 90-day supply.

GENERAL INFORMATION: You can call between 9:00 am and 4:00 pm, Pacific Time, Monday through Friday.

MEDICATIONS AVAILABLE: Amicar Injectable, Amicar Tablets, Leucovorin Calcium Injectable, Leucovorin Calcium Oral Tabs, Leukine, Methotrexate Injectable, Methotrexate Sodium Tabs, Novantrone, Thioplex

COMPANY: InterMune Pharmaceuticals

PROGRAM ADDRESS: InterMune Pharmaceuticals
                      3294 West Bayshore Road
                      Palto Alto, CA 94303

TOLL FREE PHONE NUMBER: 800-686-8036

ELIGIBILITY: You cannot have insurance that provides prescription coverage and you must be ineligible for State Medicaid. Your income has to be less than $20,150 per year ($1,679 per month). You must have a diagnosis of Chronic Granulomatous Disease.

ENROLLMENT: Anyone can call for an enrollment application form. They will send multiple copies to your doctor.

FROM YOUR DOCTOR: Your doctor will complete the application, attach a prescription (if necessary), sign the application, and mail it to InterMune Pharmaceuticals.

WHAT YOU HAVE TO DO: Stay in contact with your doctor's office. You will have to provide detailed financial and insurance information. You must sign the form.

WHERE THE MEDICATION GOES: The medication will be sent to your doctor's office. The medication will not be sent to a P.O. Box.

AMOUNT GIVEN AT ONE TIME: Usually a 90-day supply.

GENERAL INFORMATION: You can call between 9:00 am and 4:00 pm, Central Time, Monday through Friday.

MEDICATION AVAILABLE: Actimmune

COMPANY: Janssen Pharmaceutica

PROGRAM ADDRESS: Janssen Pharmaceutica
                       Patient Assistance Program
                       3rd Floor
                       1800 Robert Fulton Dr.
                       Reston, VA 22091-4346

TOLL FREE PHONE NUMBER: 800-652-6227 #2
ALTERNATIVE NUMBER: 800-526-7736

ELIGIBILITY: You cannot have insurance that provides prescription coverage and you must be ineligible for State Medicaid.

ENROLLMENT: Your doctor's office must call for the enrollment application form.

FROM YOUR DOCTOR: Your doctor will complete the application, attach a prescription (if necessary), sign the application, and mail it to Janssen Pharmaceutica.

WHAT YOU HAVE TO DO: Stay in contact with your doctor's office. You will have to provide detailed income and insurance information such as a copy of your most recent tax return or proof you did not file one. Your signature is required.

WHERE THE MEDICATION GOES: The medication will be sent to your doctor's office. The medication will not be sent to a P.O. Box.

AMOUNT GIVEN AT ONE TIME: A two (2) months' supply for Ergamisol. All medications are a one (1) month supply. Only your doctor's office can call when your supply is low.

GENERAL INFORMATION: **All medication must be for an FDA approved diagnosis.** If not, then the application will be rejected. They will not provide any medications for off-label use. You can call between 9:00 am and 5:00 pm, Eastern Time, Monday through Friday. A separate prescription is needed for Duragesic.

MEDICATIONS AVAILABLE: Cilest, Daktarin, Dipiperon, Duragesic Transdermal, Ergamisol, Fentanyl, Gyno-Daktarin, Haldol, Imap, Imodium, Impromen, Leustatin, Livostin, Motilium, Nizoral Cream, Nizoral Shampoo, Nizoral Tablets, Orap, Pancrease, Pariet, Pevaryl, Priamide, Reasec, Regranex, Reminyl, Semap, Sibelium, Sporanox Capsules, Sporanox Oral Suspension, Sporanox Injectable, Systen, Tinsel, Topamax, Vermox

COMPANY: Janssen Pharmaceutica

PROGRAM ADDRESS: Risperdal Patient Assistance Program
                           4828 Parkway Plaza Blvd.
                           Suite 220
                           Charlotte, NC 28217-1969

TOLL FREE PHONE NUMBER: 800-652-6227
FAX NUMBER: 704-357-0036

ELIGIBILITY: You cannot have insurance that provides prescription coverage and you must be ineligible for State Medicaid. There is an income limit. Income limit for a household of two (2) would be $21,000, but they do consider out-of-pocket medical expenses. Generally, income cut-off is 200% of Federal Poverty Guideline (see pg. 249-250).

ENROLLMENT: Anyone can call for an enrollment application form. Preliminary screening will be done over the phone.

FROM YOUR DOCTOR: Your doctor will complete the application, attach a prescription (if necessary), ask for quantities of 60s or 100s, sign the application, and mail it to Risperdal Patient Assistance Program.

WHAT YOU HAVE TO DO: Stay in contact with your doctor's office. You will be required to provide income and insurance information.

WHERE THE MEDICATION GOES: The medication will be sent to your doctor's office. The medication will not be sent to a P.O. Box.

AMOUNT GIVEN AT ONE TIME: Usually a 90-day supply.

GENERAL INFORMATION: Must be prescribe in quantities of 60s or 100s or will be rejected. You can call between 9:00 am and 4:00 pm, Eastern Time, Monday through Friday.

MEDICATIONS AVAILABLE: Risperdal Oral Suspension, Risperdal Tabs

COMPANY: Jones Pharmaceutical, Inc.

PROGRAM ADDRESS: Jones Pharmaceutical, Inc.
P.O. Box 46903
St. Louis, MO 63146

TOLL FREE PHONE NUMBER: 800-525-8466

ELIGIBILITY: You cannot have insurance that provides prescription coverage and you must be ineligible for State Medicaid.

ENROLLMENT: Anyone can call for an enrollment application form.

FROM YOUR DOCTOR: Your doctor will complete the application, attach a prescription (if necessary), sign the application, and mail it to Jones Pharmaceutical, Inc.

WHAT YOU HAVE TO DO: Stay in contact with your doctor's office.

WHERE THE MEDICATION GOES: The medication will be sent to your doctor's office. The medication will not be sent to a P.O. Box.

AMOUNT GIVEN AT ONE TIME: Usually a 90-day supply.

GENERAL INFORMATION: You can call between 9:00 am and 4:00 pm, Central Time, Monday through Friday.

MEDICATIONS AVAILABLE: Cytomel, Levoxyl, Tapazole

COMPANY: Key Pharmaceuticals

PROGRAM ADDRESS: Schering Labs/Key Pharmaceuticals
                        Patient Assistance Program
                        P.O. Box 52122
                        Phoenix, AZ 85072

TOLL FREE PHONE NUMBER: 800-656-9485

ELIGIBILITY: You cannot have insurance that provides prescription coverage and you must be ineligible for State Medicaid.

ENROLLMENT: Anyone can call for an enrollment application form.

FROM YOUR DOCTOR: Your doctor will complete the original application, attach a prescription (if necessary), sign the application, and mail it to Schering Labs/Key Pharmaceuticals.

WHAT YOU HAVE TO DO: Stay in contact with your doctor's office. You will have to provide detailed financial information including proof of household income. You must sign the enrollment application.

WHERE THE MEDICATION GOES: The medication will be sent to your doctor's office. The medication will not be sent to a P.O. Box.

AMOUNT GIVEN AT ONE TIME: Usually a 90-day supply.

GENERAL INFORMATION: You can call between 9:00 am and 4:00 pm, Mountain Time, Monday through Friday.

MEDICATIONS AVAILABLE: Imdur, K-Dur, Nitro-Dur, Theo-Dur ER Tablets, Trinalin Repetabs, Unid-Dur ER Tablets

COMPANY: Knoll Pharmaceutical Company

PROGRAM ADDRESS: Knoll Patient in Need Program
3000 Continental Drive, North,
Mail-Stop 4-017
Mount Olive, NJ 07828-1234

TOLL FREE PHONE NUMBER: 800-524-2474
ALTERNATIVE NUMBER: 800-240-3820

ELIGIBILITY: You cannot have insurance that provides prescription coverage and you must be ineligible for State Medicaid.

ENROLLMENT: Your doctor's office must obtain the enrollment application form by calling 800-240-3820 or *www.rxhope.com*. Knoll Pharmaceutical Co. requires your doctor to obtain either proof of income from you or a note from a social worker saying you can't afford the medication.

FROM YOUR DOCTOR: Your doctor will complete the application, attach a prescription (if necessary), sign the application, and mail it to Knoll Pharmaceutical Co.

WHAT YOU HAVE TO DO: Stay in contact with your doctor's office. You may be required to provide financial information to Knoll Pharmaceutical Co.

WHERE THE MEDICATION GOES: The medication will be sent to your doctor's office. The medication will not be sent to a P.O. Box.

AMOUNT GIVEN AT ONE TIME: Usually a 90-day supply.

GENERAL INFORMATION: You can call between 9:00 am and 4:00 pm, Eastern Time, Monday through Friday.

MEDICATIONS AVAILABLE: Isoptin SR, Isopto Carbachol, Mavik, Rythmol (only 150/300 mg), Synthroid, Tarka

COMPANY: Lederle Labs

PROGRAM ADDRESS: Lederle Labs
                        Professional Services
                        Indigent Patient Program
                        P.O. Box 8299
                        Philadelphia, PA 19101-8299

TOLL FREE PHONE NUMBER: 800-395-9938
ALTERNATIVE NUMBER: 610-688-4400

ELIGIBILITY: You cannot have insurance that provides prescription coverage and you must be ineligible for State Medicaid.

ENROLLMENT: Your doctor's office must call for an enrollment application form.

FROM YOUR DOCTOR: Your doctor will complete the application, sign the application, and mails it to Lederle Labs Professional Services Indigent Patient. A prescription is part of the application form.

WHAT YOU HAVE TO DO: Stay in contact with your doctor's office. You must sign the form.

WHERE THE MEDICATION GOES: The medication will be sent to your doctor's office. The medication will not be sent to a P.O. Box.

AMOUNT GIVEN AT ONE TIME: Usually a 90-day supply.

GENERAL INFORMATION: **No more than two (2) medications per application.** You can call between 9:00 am and 4:00 pm, Eastern Time, Monday through Friday.

MEDICATIONS AVAILABLE: Artane Elixir, Artane Tabs, Asenden, Declomycin, Diamox SR, Diamox Tabs, Loxitane, Materna, Minocin Capsules, Minocin Oral Solution, Myanbutol, Neptazane, Pyrazinamide, Rheumatrex, Suprax Oral Solution, Suprax Tabs, Zebeta, Ziac

COMPANY: Ligard Pharmaceuticals

PROGRAM ADDRESS: Ligard Assistance Program
                   10275 Science Center Drive
                   San Diego, CA 92121

TOLL FREE PHONE NUMBER: 877-654-4263
FAX NUMBER: 763-792-3266

ELIGIBILITY: You cannot have insurance that provides prescription coverage and you must be ineligible for State Medicaid.

ENROLLMENT: Your doctor's office must call for an enrollment application form. The enrollment application is sent first to you for completion. You will have to take the application form to your doctor.

FROM YOUR DOCTOR: Your doctor will complete the application, attach a prescription (if necessary), sign the application, and mail it to Ligard Assistance Program.

WHAT YOU HAVE TO DO: Stay in contact with your doctor's office. You must sign the enrollment application. You will be required to provide detailed financial and insurance information.

WHERE THE MEDICATION GOES: The medication will be sent to your doctor's office. The medication will not be sent to a P.O. Box.

AMOUNT GIVEN AT ONE TIME: Usually a 90-day supply.

GENERAL INFORMATION: You can call between 9:00 am and 5:00 pm, Eastern Time, Monday through Friday.

MEDICATIONS AVAILABLE: Ontak, Panretin Gel, Targretin Capsules, Targretin Gel

COMPANY: The Liposome Company, Inc.

PROGRAM ADDRESS: The Liposome Company, Inc.
                           Financial Assistance Program for Abelcet
                           One Research Way
                           Princeton, NJ 08540-6619

TOLL FREE PHONE NUMBER: 800-335-547

ELIGIBILITY: You cannot have insurance that provides prescription coverage and you must be ineligible for State Medicaid.

ENROLLMENT: Anyone can call for an enrollment application form.

FROM YOUR DOCTOR: Your doctor will complete the application, including a diagnosis, attach a prescription (if necessary), sign the application, and mail it to The Liposome Company, Inc.

WHAT YOU HAVE TO DO: Stay in contact with your doctor's office. You will have to provide detailed household income and insurance information.

WHERE THE MEDICATION GOES: The medication will be sent to your doctor's office, the hospital, or home health care company. The medication will not be sent to a P.O. Box.

AMOUNT GIVEN AT ONE TIME: Usually a 90-day supply.

GENERAL INFORMATION: You must be getting Abelcet from a hospital, physician, or home health care company for a **"medically appropriate application."** This is a replacement program. You can call between 9:00 am and 4:00 pm, Eastern Time, Monday through Friday.

MEDICATION AVAILABLE: Abelcet

COMPANY:　　　　　　　Mead Johnson and Company

PROGRAM ADDRESS:　Mead Johnson
　　　　　　　　　　　Nutritional Infant Division
　　　　　　　　　　　Helping Hands
　　　　　　　　　　　2400 W. Lloyd Expressway
　　　　　　　　　　　Evansville, IN 47721

TOLL FREE PHONE NUMBER:　800-222-9123
ALTERNATIVE NUMBER:　　　812-429-5000

ELIGIBILITY: You cannot have insurance that provides prescription coverage and you must be ineligible for State Medicaid. This program is for infants under one year of age.

ENROLLMENT: Your doctor's office should call and explain your circumstances.

FROM YOUR DOCTOR: The doctor calls the sales representative who will determine if the family qualifies for assistance.

WHAT YOU HAVE TO DO: Stay in contact with your doctor's office. Tell your doctor you can't afford the formula.

WHERE THE MEDICATION GOES: Usually sent directly to the family.

AMOUNT GIVEN AT ONE TIME: Usually a 90-day supply.

GENERAL INFORMATION: You can call between 9:00 am and 4:00 pm, Central Time, Monday through Friday.

MEDICATIONS AVAILABLE: Metabolic Formulas, Nutramigen, Pregestimil

COMPANY: Medeva Pharmaceuticals, Inc.

PROGRAM ADDRESS: Medeva Pharmaceuticals, Inc.
                         P.O. Box 31766
                         Rochester, NY 14603

TOLL FREE PHONE NUMBER: 800-234-5535 x5220
FAX NUMBER: 716-272-3935

ELIGIBILITY: You cannot have insurance that provides prescription coverage and you must be ineligible for State Medicaid. Your household income must be below $8,860 per year ($738 per month) for a single person; for a household of two (2) income must be below $12,500 per year ($1,040 per month).

ENROLLMENT: Anyone can call for an enrollment application form. The enrollment application form will be sent directly to your doctor.

FROM YOUR DOCTOR: Your doctor will complete the application, attach a prescription (if necessary), sign the application, and mail it to Medeva Pharmaceuticals, Inc.

WHAT YOU HAVE TO DO: Stay in contact with your doctor's office. You must sign the enrollment application form.

WHERE THE MEDICATION GOES: The medication will be sent to your doctor's office. The medication will not be sent to a P.O. Box.

AMOUNT GIVEN AT ONE TIME: Usually a 90-day supply.

GENERAL INFORMATION: You can call between 9:00 am and 4:00 pm, Eastern Time, Monday through Friday.

MEDICATIONS AVAILABLE: Delsym Extended Release, Gastrocrom Oral Concentrate, Hylorel, Mykrox, Pediapred Oral Solution, Semprex-D, Velstar Intravesical Solution, Zaroxolyn

COMPANY: Medicis Pharmaceutical Corp.

PROGRAM ADDRESS: Medicis Pharmaceutical Corp.
4343 Camelback Rd.
Phoenix, AZ 85018

TOLL FREE PHONE NUMBER: 800-533-3376

ELIGIBILITY: You cannot have insurance that provides prescription coverage and you must be ineligible for State Medicaid.

ENROLLMENT: Your doctor's office needs to call for an enrollment application form.

FROM YOUR DOCTOR: Your doctor needs to write a letter on office stationery including diagnosis, lack of insurance, financial hardship, attach a prescription, sign the letter, and mail it to Medicis Pharmaceutical Corp.

WHAT YOU HAVE TO DO: Stay in contact with your doctor's office.

WHERE THE MEDICATION GOES: The medication will be sent to your doctor's office. The medication will not be sent to a P.O. Box.

AMOUNT GIVEN AT ONE TIME: Usually a 90-day supply.

GENERAL INFORMATION: You can call between 9:00 am and 4:00 pm, Mountain Time, Monday through Friday.

MEDICATIONS AVAILABLE: Benzashave Cream, Dynacin Capsules, Synalar Cream, Synalar Ointment, Theramycin Topical Solution, Triaz Cleanser, Triaz Gel, Zonalon Cream

COMPANY: Medimmune, Inc.

PROGRAM ADDRESS: Synagis Secure Program
                                      P.O. Box 222197
                                      Charlotte, NC 28222-2197

TOLL FREE PHONE NUMBER: 877-480-8082
ALTERNATIVE NUMBER: 877-633-4411
FAX NUMBER: 877-675-6513

ELIGIBILITY: You cannot have insurance that provides prescription coverage and you must be ineligible for State Medicaid.

ENROLLMENT: Your doctor or the hospital must call for an enrollment application form. Synagis Secure Program will fax an application and program information. The information for the application can be taken over the phone or from the application.

FROM YOUR DOCTOR: Your doctor or hospital representative will complete the application, attach a prescription (if necessary), sign the application, and mail or fax it to Synagis Secure Program.

WHAT YOU HAVE TO DO: Stay in contact with your doctor's office. You will have to provide detailed income and insurance information. You must sign the enrollment application.

WHERE THE MEDICATION GOES: Replacements are provided to the hospital or physician.

GENERAL INFORMATION: You can call between 9:00 am and 4:00 pm, Eastern Time, Monday through Friday.

MEDICATION AVAILABLE: Synagis

COMPANY: Merck & Company

PROGRAM ADDRESS: Merck Patient Assistance Program
                            P.O. Box 2230
                            Pittsburgh, PA 19486-0004

TOLL FREE PHONE NUMBER: 800-994-2111
                            (Automatic line for doctors)
ALTERNATIVE NUMBER: 800-999-1796

ELIGIBILITY: You cannot have insurance that provides prescription coverage and you must be ineligible for State Medicaid.

ENROLLMENT: Merck wants only the doctor's office to call for an enrollment application form.

FROM YOUR DOCTOR: Your doctor will complete the application, attach a prescription (if necessary), sign the application, and mail it to Merck Patient Assistance Program.

WHAT YOU HAVE TO DO: Stay in contact with your doctor's office. You will have to provide detailed financial and insurance information. You will have to sign the enrollment application.

WHERE THE MEDICATION GOES: The medication will be sent to your doctor's office. The medication will not be sent to a P.O. Box.

AMOUNT GIVEN AT ONE TIME: Usually a 90-day supply.

GENERAL INFORMATION: They have an easy program for the doctor's office staff to use. Simply call the 800 number and enter the doctor's DEA number. Call the second 800 number if there are any problems or questions. Merck will only accept their own application in their own return envelopes. Their program includes all the oral medicines and injectable chemotherapeutics. You can call between 9:00 am and 4:00 pm, Eastern Time, Monday through Friday.

MEDICATIONS AVAILABLE: Aldoclor, Aldomet, Blocadren, Chibroxin, Clinoril, Cogentin Injectable, Cogentin Tabs, Cosmegin, Cozaar, Cuprimine, Daranide, Decadron Elixir, Decadron LA Sterile Suspension, Decadron Phosphate Sterile Ophthalmic Ointment, Decadron Phosphate Sterile Ophthalmic Solution, Decadron Phosphate Injection, Decadron Tabs, Demser, Diuril Capsules, Diuril Oral Suspension, Diuril Tabs, Dolobid, Edecrin, Elspar, Flexeril, Fosamax, Humorsol, Hydrocortone Tabs, HydroDIURIL, Hyzaar, Indocin Oral Suspension, Indocin SR Capsules, Indocin Suppositories, Lacrisert, Maxalt, Mephyton, Mevacor, Mintezol Chewable Tabs, Mintezol Oral Suspension, Moduretic, Mustargen, Neodecadron Ophthalmic Ointment, Pepcid Tabs, Pepcid RPD, Pepcid Oral Suspension, Periactin Tabs, Periactin Syrup, Primaxin, Prinivil, Prinizide, Propecia, Proscar, Singulair Chewable Tabs, Singulair Tabs, Syprine, Timolide, Timoptic, Timoptic XE, Timoptic in Ocudose, Timoptic Ophthalmic Gel, Trusopt Ophthalmic Solution, Urecholine, Vaseretic, Vasotec, Vioxx, Vivactil, Zocor

COMPANY: Merck & Company

PROGRAM ADDRESS: Merck Patient Assistance Program
                              Aggrastat Assistance Program
                              P.O. Box 222137
                              Charlotte, NC 28222-2137

TOLL FREE PHONE NUMBER: 877-810-0595

ELIGIBILITY: You cannot have insurance that provides prescription coverage and you must be ineligible for State Medicaid.

ENROLLMENT: The hospital must call to get an enrollment application. The original form may be copied. The caller must have the hospital's DEA number, a contact person's name (usually a social worker), and the hospital's address. The application is faxed to the hospital.

FROM YOUR DOCTOR: Your doctor's name must be on the application. A hospital representative (usually a social worker) must sign the enrollment application, include the pharmacy dispensing record, drug invoice (must be included) and mail it to Merck Patient Assistance Program for Aggrastat.

WHAT YOU HAVE TO DO: You will have to provide detailed household financial information and proof of insurance, if any.

WHERE THE MEDICATION GOES: Sent to the hospital pharmacy.

AMOUNT GIVEN AT ONE TIME: Replacement amount only.

GENERAL INFORMATION: It's a product replacement program. You can call between 9:00 am and 4:00 pm, Eastern Time, Monday through Friday.

MEDICATIONS AVAILABLE: Aggrastat Injectable, Aggrastat Premix Injectable

COMPANY: Merck & Company

PROGRAM ADDRESS: Crixivan Patient Assistance Services
                        SUPPORT P.O. Box 222137
                        Charlotte, NC 28222-2137

TOLL FREE PHONE NUMBER: 800-850-3430
FAX NUMBER: 704-357-0036

ELIGIBILITY: You cannot have insurance that provides prescription coverage and you must be ineligible for State Medicaid.

ENROLLMENT: Your doctor's office should call and request an enrollment application form. Merck will fax your doctor the form. This form can be copied.

FROM YOUR DOCTOR: Your doctor will complete the application, attach a prescription (if necessary), sign the application, and mail it to Crixivan Patient Assistance Services.

WHAT YOU HAVE TO DO: Stay in contact with your doctor's office. You will have to provide detailed financial and insurance information.

WHERE THE MEDICATION GOES: The medication will be sent to your doctor's office. The medication will not be sent to a P.O. Box.

AMOUNT GIVEN AT ONE TIME: Usually a 90-day supply.

GENERAL INFORMATION: This is a completely separate program for this AIDS/HIV medication. This program uses a different form and procedure. The approved application is good for a year of medication without having to reapply. Merck will let physician know when a new Rx is needed. You can call between 9:00 am and 4:00 pm, Eastern Time, Monday through Friday.

MEDICATION AVAILABLE: Crixivan

COMPANY: MGI Pharmaceutical, Inc.

PROGRAM ADDRESS: MGI Pharmaceutical, Inc.
Salagen Tablets PAP
1101 King Street, Suite 600
Alexandria VA 22314

TOLL FREE PHONE NUMBER: 888-743-5711
FAX NUMBER: 703-535-5027

ELIGIBILITY: You cannot have insurance that provides prescription coverage and you must be ineligible for State Medicaid.

ENROLLMENT: Anyone can call for an enrollment application form. But, have your doctor call since MGI Pharmaceutical, Inc., requires the doctor's DEA number at the time of enrollment.

FROM YOUR DOCTOR: Your doctor will complete the application, attach a prescription (if necessary), sign the application, and mail it to MGI Pharmaceutical, Inc.

WHAT YOU HAVE TO DO: Stay in contact with your doctor's office. You will have to provide detailed financial and insurance information.

WHERE THE MEDICATION GOES: The medication will be sent to your doctor's office. The medication will not be sent to a P.O. Box.

AMOUNT GIVEN AT ONE TIME: Usually a 90-day supply.

GENERAL INFORMATION: You can call between 9:00 am and 4:00 pm, Eastern Time, Monday through Friday.

MEDICATION AVAILABLE: Salagen

COMPANY: Monarch Pharmaceuticals

PROGRAM ADDRESS: Monarch Pharmaceuticals
                           355 Beecham St.
                           Bristol, TN 37620

TOLL FREE PHONE NUMBER: 800-776-3637
FAX NUMBER: 423-989-6279

ELIGIBILITY: You cannot have insurance that provides prescription coverage and you must be ineligible for State Medicaid.

ENROLLMENT: Your doctor must call for an enrollment application form.

FROM YOUR DOCTOR: Your doctor will complete the application, attach a prescription (if necessary), sign the application, and mail it to Monarch Pharmaceuticals.

WHAT YOU HAVE TO DO: Stay in contact with your doctor's office.

WHERE THE MEDICATION GOES: The medication will be sent to your doctor's office. The medication will not be sent to a P.O. Box.

AMOUNT GIVEN AT ONE TIME: Usually a 90-day supply.

GENERAL INFORMATION: You can call between 9:00 am and 5:00 pm, Eastern Time, Monday through Friday.

MEDICATIONS AVAILABLE: Altace, Anusol-HC 2.5% Cream, Anusol-HC 25 mg Suppositories, Cortisporin Ophthalmic Ointment, Cortisporin Ophthalmic Suspension, Cortisporin Optic Ointment, Cortisporin Optic Solution, Cortisporin Optic Suspension, Cortisporin Optic TC Suspension, Kemadrin, Menest 0.3 mg Capsules, Menest 0.625 mg Capsules, Menest 1.25 mg Capsules, Menest 2.5 mg Tabs, Neosporin GU, Neosporin Ophthalmic Ointment, Neosporin Ophthalmic Solution, Pediotic Ophthalmic Suspension, Polysporin Ophthalmic Ointment, Procanbid 100 mg Tabs, Procanbid 500 mg Tabs, Proctocort 1% Cream, Proctocort 30 mg Suppositories, Proloprim 100 mg Tabs, Proloprim 500 mg. Tabs, Quibron, Septra 80 mg Tabs, Septra DS 160 mg Tabs, Septra Suspension, Silvadene 1% Cream, Thalitone 15 mg Tabs, Thalitone 25 mg Tabs, Vira-A Ophthalmic Ointment, Viroptic 1% Ophthalmic Solution

COMPANY: MS Pathways

PROGRAM ADDRESS: The Betaseron Foundation
                        4828 Parkway Plaza Blvd., Suite 220
                        Charlotte, NC 28217-1969

TOLL FREE PHONE NUMBER: 800-948-5777
FAX NUMBER: 704-357-0036

ELIGIBILITY: You cannot have insurance that provides prescription coverage and you must be ineligible for State Medicaid. You must have a diagnosis of Remitting/Relapsing Multiple Sclerosis (MS) and be a U.S. resident. Your income must be below $20,000 per year ($1,666 per month).

ENROLLMENT: Anyone can call for an enrollment application form.

FROM YOUR DOCTOR: Your doctor will complete the application, attach a prescription (if necessary), sign the application, and mail it to The Betaseron Foundation.

WHAT YOU HAVE TO DO: Stay in contact with your doctor's office. You will have to provide detailed financial and insurance information. You must sign the enrollment application.

WHERE THE MEDICATION GOES: You will receive a plastic card (like a credit card) and instructions for your pharmacy.

AMOUNT GIVEN AT ONE TIME: Twelve (12), 30-day supply.

GENERAL INFORMATION: You can call between 9:00 am and 5:00 pm, Eastern Time, Monday through Friday. If you have no insurance with an income between $20,000-$50,000, you may qualify for a price reduction program.

MEDICATION AVAILABLE: Betaseron

COMPANY: Muro Pharmaceutical, Inc.

PROGRAM ADDRESS: Muro Pharmaceutical, Inc.
                        890 East Street
                        Tweksbury, MA 01876-1496

TOLL FREE PHONE NUMBER: 800-225-0974, option 3
ALTERNATIVE NUMBER: 978-851-5981
FAX NUMBER: 978-851-7346

ELIGIBILITY: You cannot have insurance that provides prescription coverage and you must be ineligible for State Medicaid.

ENROLLMENT: Anyone can call for an enrollment application form.

FROM YOUR DOCTOR: Your doctor will complete the application, attach a prescription (if necessary), sign the application, and mail it to Muro Pharmaceutical, Inc.

WHAT YOU HAVE TO DO: Stay in contact with your doctor's office. You must sign the enrollment application form.

WHERE THE MEDICATION GOES: The medication will be sent to your doctor's office. The medication will not be sent to a P.O. Box.

AMOUNT GIVEN AT ONE TIME: A maximum of 6 months.

GENERAL INFORMATION: If you have been denied for Medicaid, a copy of the denial letter must be attached. You can call between 9:00 am and 4:00 pm, Eastern Time, Monday through Friday.

MEDICATIONS AVAILABLE: Prelone Syrup, Volmax ER Tabs

PROGRAM ADDRESS: NABI Reimbursement Support Program
8990 Springbrook Dr.
Suite 200
Minneapolis, MN 55433

TOLL FREE PHONE NUMBER: 800-789-2099

ELIGIBILITY: You cannot have insurance that provides prescription coverage and you must be ineligible for State Medicaid.

ENROLLMENT: Your doctor's office must call for an enrollment application form.

FROM YOUR DOCTOR: Your doctor will complete the application, attach a prescription (if necessary), sign the application, and mail it to NABI Reimbursement Support Program.

WHAT YOU HAVE TO DO: Stay in contact with your doctor's office. You will have to provide detailed financial and insurance information. You must sign the enrollment application.

WHERE THE MEDICATION GOES: The medication will be sent to your doctor's office. The medication will not be sent to a P.O. Box.

AMOUNT GIVEN AT ONE TIME: Usually a 90-day supply.

GENERAL INFORMATION: You can call between 9:00 am and 4:00 pm, Central Time, Monday through Friday.

MEDICATION AVAILABLE: Win Rho SDF

PROGRAM ADDRESS: National Organization for Rare Diseases
(NORD)
Patient Assistance Programs
P.O. Box 8923
New Fairfield, CT 06812-8923

TOLL FREE PHONE NUMBER: 800-999-6673
ALTERNATIVE NUMBER: 888-628-6673
FAX NUMBER: 203-746-6896

ELIGIBILITY: You cannot have insurance that provides prescription coverage and you must be ineligible for State Medicaid.

ENROLLMENT: Anyone can call for an enrollment application form.

FROM YOUR DOCTOR: Your doctor will complete the application, attach a prescription (if necessary), sign the application, and mail it to National Organization for Rare Diseases (NORD).

WHAT YOU HAVE TO DO: Stay in contact with your doctor's office. You will have to provide detailed financial and insurance information. Some of the medication will require proof of household income. You must sign the enrollment application form.

WHERE THE MEDICATION GOES: Some medication will be sent to your doctor's office. Some medication will require you to pay a handling fee from a mail-order pharmacy.

AMOUNT GIVEN AT ONE TIME: Usually a 90-day supply.

GENERAL INFORMATION: NORD administers a number of different programs for investigational and approved pharmaceutical products manufactured for a number of pharmaceutical companies. NORD is a federation of voluntary health organizations committed to supporting and treating those with rare diseases. NORD determines how much of the monthly cost you can afford to pay. NORD will usually pay 25% to 100% of the monthly cost. You can call between 9:00 am and 4:00 pm, Eastern Time, Monday through Friday.

Special phone numbers to use for specific medications:

Acthar Gel:	800-459-7599
Biphenyl:	800-711-0811
Copaxone:	800-887-8100
Menomune:	877-798-8716
Provigil:	800-675-8415
Rilutek:	800-459-7599
Serostim:	888-628-6673
Sucraid:	888-867-7526
Xyrem:	888-867-7526

MEDICATIONS AVAILABLE: Acthar Gel, Botox, Buphenyl, Busulfex, Carnitor, Copaxone, Cystadane, ITB, Matulane, Menomune, Provigil, Rilutek, Serostim, Sucraid, Urea Cycle Therapy, Xyrem

COMPANY: Novartis Pharmaceuticals

PROGRAM ADDRESS: Novartis Patient Assistance Program
                      P.O. Box 52052
                      Phoenix, AZ 85072-0170

TOLL FREE PHONE NUMBER: 800-257-3273
ALTERNATIVE NUMBER: 888-455-6655
FAX NUMBER: 908-277-4399

ELIGIBILITY: You cannot have insurance that provides prescription coverage and you must be ineligible for State Medicaid.

ENROLLMENT: Anyone can call for an enrollment application form. Whoever calls will need the doctor's name, the prescription information, your income and medical expense information, and whether or not you receive benefits from insurance, Medicaid, VA, or anyone else.

FROM YOUR DOCTOR: Your doctor will complete the application, attach a prescription (if necessary), sign the application, and mail it to Novartis Patient Assistance Program. Your doctor will also give you a prescription to take to the pharmacy.

WHAT YOU HAVE TO DO: Stay in contact with your doctor's office. You will have to provide detailed financial and insurance information, including proof of patient/household income. You must sign the enrollment application.

WHERE THE MEDICATION GOES: Novartis Patient Assistance Program will send a card to your doctor. The doctor will give it to you. This card will act like a **"charge card"** at the pharmacy.

AMOUNT GIVEN AT ONE TIME: You will be given a number for the pharmacy to call for the initial 30-day supply when you call to register. Once the application is received, another 60 days is authorized.

GENERAL INFORMATION: You can call between 9:00 am and 8:00 pm, Eastern Time, Monday through Friday. Each medication has different income guidelines. They enter your information into their computer, which determines eligibility. The guidelines are liberal. If the Novartis medication the patient needs isn't covered, it's a good idea to write a letter of appeal to the program; they may consider providing coverage for the medication.

MEDICATIONS AVAILABLE: Aredia, Clozaril, Comtan, Desferal, Diovan Capsules, Diovan HCT, Exelon, Femara, Lamisil 1.0% Solution, Lamprene, Lescol, Lotensin, Lotensin HCT, Lotrel, Metopirone Capsules, Miacalcin, Migranal Nasal Spray, Neoral Capsules, Neoral Oral Suspension, Sandimmune, Sandostatin, Sandostatin LAR Depot, Starlix, Tegretol Chewable Tabs, Tegretol XR Tabs, Tegretol PM Capsules, Tegretol Oral Suspension, Trilaptal, Voltaren Tabs, Voltaren XR

COMPANY: Novartis Pharmaceuticals

PROGRAM ADDRESS: Sandoz Pharmaceuticals Corp.
                    59 Route 10
                    East Hanover, NJ 07936

TOLL FREE PHONE NUMBER: 800-447-6673
ALTERNATIVE NUMBER: 888-455-6655

ELIGIBILITY: You cannot have insurance that provides prescription coverage and you must be ineligible for State Medicaid.

ENROLLMENT: Anyone can call for an enrollment application form.

FROM YOUR DOCTOR: Your doctor will complete the application, attach a prescription (if necessary), sign the application, and mail it to Sandoz Pharmaceuticals Corp.

WHAT YOU HAVE TO DO: Stay in contact with your doctor's office. You may have to provide financial and insurance information.

WHERE THE MEDICATION GOES: The medication will be sent to your doctor's office. The medication will not be sent to a P.O. Box.

AMOUNT GIVEN AT ONE TIME: Usually a 90-day supply.

GENERAL INFORMATION: You can call between 9:00 am and 4:00 pm, Eastern Time, Monday through Friday.

MEDICATIONS AVAILABLE: Clozaril, Neoral Capsules, Parlodel Capsules, Parlodel Tabs, Sandimmune Capsules, Sandimmune Oral Suspension, Sandoglobulin, Sandostatin

COMPANY: Novo-Nordisk Pharmaceuticals, Inc.

PROGRAM ADDRESS: Novo-Nordisk Pharmaceuticals, Inc.
                            Attn. Indigent Program Administrator
                            100 Overlook Center, Suite 200
                            Princeton, NJ 08540-7810

TOLL FREE PHONE NUMBER: 800-727-6500
ALTERNATE PHONE NUMBER   609-987-5800
FAX NUMBER: 609-987-3092

ELIGIBILITY: You cannot have insurance that provides prescription coverage and you must be ineligible for State Medicaid.

ENROLLMENT: Anyone can call for an enrollment application form.

FROM YOUR DOCTOR: Your doctor will complete the application, attach a prescription (if necessary), sign the application, and mail it to Novo-Nordisk Pharmaceuticals, Inc.

WHAT YOU HAVE TO DO: Stay in contact with your doctor's office. You may have to provide financial and insurance information.

WHERE THE MEDICATION GOES: The medication will be sent to your doctor's office. The medication will not be sent to a P.O. Box.

AMOUNT GIVEN AT ONE TIME: Usually a 90-day supply.

GENERAL INFORMATION: You can call between 9:00 am and 4:00 pm, Eastern Time, Monday through Friday.

MEDICATIONS AVAILABLE: Novolin Novopen III, Novolin Novopen IV, Novolin Novopen V, Prandin 0.05 mg Tabs, Prandin 1.0 mg Tabs, Prandin 2.0 mg Tabs, Velosulin BR

COMPANY: Oclassen Dermatologics, Inc.

PROGRAM ADDRESS: Oclassen Dermatologics, Inc.
                            311 Bonnie Circle
                            P.O. Box 1900
                            Corona, CA 92878

TOLL FREE PHONE NUMBER: 800-272-5525

ELIGIBILITY: You cannot have insurance that provides prescription coverage and you must be ineligible for State Medicaid.

ENROLLMENT: There is no formal program. Your doctor's office should call and start the enrollment.

FROM YOUR DOCTOR: Your doctor will have to write a letter on office letterhead stationery stating your medical need and a lack of prescription coverage. Your doctor will have to attach a prescription, and mail it to Oclassen Dermatologics, Inc.

WHAT YOU HAVE TO DO: Stay in contact with your doctor's office. You may have to provide financial and insurance information.

WHERE THE MEDICATION GOES: The medication will be sent to your doctor's office. The medication will not be sent to a P.O. Box.

AMOUNT GIVEN AT ONE TIME: Usually a 90-day supply.

GENERAL INFORMATION: Oclassen Dermatologics, Inc., may help if you can show a medical need and you cannot afford the medication. You can call between 9:00 am and 4:00 pm, Pacific Time, Monday through Friday.

MEDICATIONS AVAILABLE: Cinobac, Condylox Gel, Condylox Solution, Cordran Cream, Cordran Lotion, Cordran Ointment, Cordran Tape, Cormax Ointment, Cormax Scalp Application, Monodox

COMPANY: Organon, Inc.

PROGRAM ADDRESS: Organon, Inc.
375 Mount Pleasant Ave.
West Orange, NJ 07052

TOLL FREE PHONE NUMBER: 800-631-1253
ALTERNATIVE NUMBER: 973-325-4896

ELIGIBILITY: You cannot have insurance that provides prescription coverage and you must be ineligible for State Medicaid.

ENROLLMENT: Your doctor's office needs to call Organon, Inc. They will send their sales representative out to your doctor's office to go over the form with your doctor.

FROM YOUR DOCTOR: Your doctor will complete the application, attach a prescription (if necessary), sign the application, and mail it to Organon, Inc.

WHAT YOU HAVE TO DO: Stay in contact with your doctor's office.

WHERE THE MEDICATION GOES: The medication will be sent to your doctor's office. The medication will not be sent to a P.O. Box.

AMOUNT GIVEN AT ONE TIME: Usually a 90-day supply.

GENERAL INFORMATION: You can call between 9:00 am and 4:00 pm, Eastern Time, Monday through Friday.

MEDICATION AVAILABLE: Remeron

COMPANY: Ortho-McNeil Pharmaceuticals

PROGRAM ADDRESS: Ortho-McNeil Pharmaceuticals
                              Patient Assistant Program
                              1800 Robert Fulton Dr.
                              3rd Floor
                              Reston, VA 20191

TOLL FREE PHONE NUMBER: 800-797-7737

ELIGIBILITY: You cannot have insurance that provides prescription coverage and you must be ineligible for State Medicaid.

ENROLLMENT: Anyone can call for an enrollment application form but you should have your doctor's office call. At the time of enrollment Ortho-McNeil will need your name, social security number, date of birth, your doctor's name, their DEA number, address, phone number, and the medication and dose. The applications are medication specific. The form is sent directly your doctor.

FROM YOUR DOCTOR: Your doctor will complete the application, attach a prescription (if necessary), sign the application, and give the enrollment application back to you to complete.

WHAT YOU HAVE TO DO: Stay in contact with your doctor's office. **You must call the company and review the application before you mail it to Ortho-McNeil Pharmaceuticals.**

WHERE THE MEDICATION GOES: The medication will be sent to your doctor's office. The medication will not be sent to a P.O. Box.

AMOUNT GIVEN AT ONE TIME: Usually a 90-day supply.

GENERAL INFORMATION: You can call between 9:00 am and 5:00 pm, Eastern Time, Monday through Friday.

MEDICATIONS AVAILABLE ACI-Jel, Erycette Topical Solution, Floxin, Grifulvin V Tabs, Haldol, Haldol Decanoate Injectable 50 mg/ml, Haldol Decanoate Injectable 100 mg/ml, Leustain, Levaquin, Micronor, Modicon, Monistat-3, Monistat Derm, Ortho-Cept, Ortho-Cyclen, Ortho-Dienestrol, Ortho-Est, Ortho-Novum, Ortho-Tri-Cyclen, Pancrease Capsules, Pancrease MT Capsules, Paraflex, Parafon Forte, Poltolectin, Retin A, Spectazole, Sultrin, Terazol, Tylenol with Codeine (All Forms), Tylox, Ultram, Vascor

COMPANY: Ortho-McNeil Pharmaceuticals

PROGRAM ADDRESS: Ortho-McNeil Pharmaceuticals
                           Regranex Patient Assistance Program
                           P.O. Box 938
                           Somerville, NJ 08876

TOLL FREE PHONE NUMBER: 888-734-7263
ALTERNATIVE NUMBER: 800-797-7737 #1

ELIGIBILITY: You cannot have insurance that provides prescription coverage and you must be ineligible for State Medicaid.

ENROLLMENT: Your doctor's office must call to register you by phone. The enrollment application form will be mailed or faxed to your doctor's office.

FROM YOUR DOCTOR: Your doctor will complete the application, attach a prescription (which has to include their DEA number), sign the application, and return the enrollment application back to you.

WHAT YOU HAVE TO DO: Stay in contact with your doctor's office. You will have to provide financial and insurance information. You will have to sign the form and mail it to Regranex Patient Assistance Program.

WHERE THE MEDICATION GOES: The medication will be sent to your doctor's office. The medication will not be sent to a P.O. Box.

AMOUNT GIVEN AT ONE TIME: One tube of Regranex will be shipped at a time, up to six tubes for a course of treatment. You may receive two treatment courses per year.

GENERAL INFORMATION: You can call between 8:30 am and 5:00 Eastern Time, Monday through Friday. **This is truly a program of last resort.**

MEDICATION AVAILABLE: Regranex Gel

COMPANY: Ortho-McNeil Pharmaceuticals

PROGRAM ADDRESS: Ortho-Biotech, Inc.
                        Patient Assistant Program
                        1800 Robert Fulton Dr.
                        3rd Floor
                        Reston, VA 20191

TOLL FREE PHONE NUMBER: 800-553-3851

ELIGIBILITY: You cannot have insurance that provides prescription coverage and you must be ineligible for State Medicaid.

ENROLLMENT: Your doctor's office must call for an enrollment application form. Your doctor will need financial and insurance information at the time of the call.

FROM YOUR DOCTOR: Your doctor will complete the application, attach a prescription (if necessary), sign the application, and mail it to Ortho-Biotech, Inc.

WHAT YOU HAVE TO DO: Stay in contact with your doctor's office. You will have to provide detailed financial and insurance information.

WHERE THE MEDICATION GOES: The medication will be sent to your doctor's office. The medication will not be sent to a P.O. Box.

AMOUNT GIVEN AT ONE TIME: Usually a 90-day supply.

GENERAL INFORMATION: Medicare covers Procrit if it is given to you in the doctor's office. Ortho-Biotech, Inc., would like your doctor to not charge a fee. You can call between 9:00 am and 4:00 pm, Eastern Time, Monday through Friday.

MEDICATIONS AVAILABLE: Leustatin, Procrit

COMPANY: Paddock Laboratories, Inc.

PROGRAM ADDRESS: Paddock Laboratories, Inc.
3950 Quebec Ave., North
Minneapolis, MN 55427

TOLL FREE PHONE NUMBER: 800-328-5113

ELIGIBILITY: You cannot have insurance that provides prescription coverage and you must be ineligible for State Medicaid.

ENROLLMENT: Anyone can call for an enrollment application form.

FROM YOUR DOCTOR: Your doctor will complete the application, attach a prescription (if necessary), sign the application, and mail it to Paddock Laboratories, Inc.

WHAT YOU HAVE TO DO: Stay in contact with your doctor's office. You may have to provide financial and insurance information.

WHERE THE MEDICATION GOES: The medication will be sent to your doctor's office. The medication will not be sent to a P.O. Box.

AMOUNT GIVEN AT ONE TIME: Usually a 90-day supply.

GENERAL INFORMATION: You can call between 9:00 am and 4:00 pm, Central Time, Monday through Friday.

MEDICATION AVAILABLE: Viokase

COMPANY: Par Pharmaceuticals, Inc.

PROGRAM ADDRESS: Par Pharmaceuticals, Inc.
Customer Service-Indigent Program
One Ram Ridge Rd.
Spring Valley, NY 10977

TOLL FREE PHONE NUMBER: 800-828-9393 ext. 774
ALTERNATIVE NUMBER: 914-425-7100

ELIGIBILITY: You cannot have insurance that provides prescription coverage and you must be ineligible for State Medicaid.

ENROLLMENT: Anyone can call for an enrollment application form. The enroll application form will only be sent to your doctor's office.

FROM YOUR DOCTOR: Your doctor will complete the application, attach a prescription (if necessary), sign the application, enclose a copy of their DEA license, and mail it to Par Pharmaceuticals, Inc.

WHAT YOU HAVE TO DO: Stay in contact with your doctor's office. You may have to provide financial and insurance information.

WHERE THE MEDICATION GOES: The medication will be sent to your doctor's office. The medication will not be sent to a P.O. Box.

AMOUNT GIVEN AT ONE TIME: Usually a 90-day supply.

GENERAL INFORMATION: You can call between 9:00 am and 4:00 pm, Eastern Time, Monday through Friday.

MEDICATIONS AVAILABLE: Capoten, Zovirax

COMPANY: Pasteur Merieux Connaught

PROGRAM ADDRESS: Pasteur Indigent Patient Program
                            Route 611,
                            Discovery Drive
                            Swiftwater, PA 18370-0187

TOLL FREE PHONE NUMBER: 800-822-2463

ELIGIBILITY: You cannot have insurance that provides prescription coverage and you must be ineligible for State Medicaid. Eligibility is determined on a case-by-case basis. Your household income must be below the Federal Poverty Guideline (see pg. 249-250). You must be a U.S. resident.

ENROLLMENT: Your doctor's office must call for an enrollment application.

FROM YOUR DOCTOR: Your doctor will complete the application, attach a prescription, sign the application, and mail it to Pasteur Indigent Patient Program. Your doctor must agree not to charge you for treatment related to these products or to receive any payment for these products. For rabies vaccines, specified dosages are needed along with the patient's age and weight.

WHAT YOU HAVE TO DO: Stay in contact with your doctor's office.

WHERE THE MEDICATION GOES: The medication will be sent to your doctor's office. The medication will not be sent to a P.O. Box.

AMOUNT GIVEN AT ONE TIME: 6 doses of TheraCys to start the treatment. A patient may receive 11 doses (total, 6 for start-up, 5 for maintenance doses). Imovax and Imogam as prescribed in ml. A single dose of Menomune is provided.

GENERAL INFORMATION: You can call between 9:00 am and 4:00 pm, Eastern Time, Monday through Friday.

MEDICATIONS AVAILABLE: Imogam, Imogam HT, Imovax, TheraCys BCG

COMPANY: Parke-Davis

PROGRAM ADDRESS: Warner-Lambert
                            Patient Assistance Program
                            P.O. Box 1058
                            Somerville, NJ 08876

TOLL FREE PHONE NUMBER: 800-223-0432, #4
ALTERNATIVE NUMBER: 908-725-1247
FAX NUMBER: 908-707-9544

ELIGIBILITY: You cannot have insurance that provides prescription coverage and you must be ineligible for State Medicaid. Income limit for a single household is under $16,000 per year ($1,333 per month), for a family (undefined) is under $25,000 ($2,082 per month).

ENROLLMENT: Your doctor's office should contact their Parke-Davis representative for an enrollment application.

FROM YOUR DOCTOR: Your doctor will complete the application, attach a prescription (including their DEA number), signs the application and mail it to Parke-Davis.

WHAT YOU HAVE TO DO: Stay in contact with your doctor's office. You will need to provide financial and insurance information.

WHERE THE MEDICATION GOES: The medication will be sent to your doctor's office. The medication will not be sent to a P.O. Box.

AMOUNT GIVEN AT ONE TIME: Usually a 90-day supply.

GENERAL INFORMATION: You can call between 8:30 am and 5:00 pm, Eastern Time, Monday through Friday.

MEDICATIONS AVAILABLE: Accupril, Accuretic, Cerebyx, Dilantin 21 Tabs, Dilantin 125 Syrup, Dilantin Fe Tabs, Dilantin Infatabs, Dilantin Kapseals, Estrostep, FemHRT, Lipitor, Loestrin, Neurontin, Zarontin Capsules, Zarontin Syrup

COMPANY: PathoGenesis Corporation

PROGRAM ADDRESS: TOBI Patient Support Program
                        5215 Old Orchard Rd.
                        Suite 900
                        Skokie, IL 60077

TOLL FREE PHONE NUMBER: 888-508-8624
FAX NUMBER: 847-583-5459

ELIGIBILITY: You cannot have insurance that provides prescription coverage and you must be ineligible for State Medicaid. You must have a diagnosis of Cystic Fibrosis. You must be a permanent U.S. resident.

ENROLLMENT: Your doctor's office should call for an enrollment application form. The application will be sent to your doctor's office.

FROM YOUR DOCTOR: Your doctor will complete the enrollment application, attach a prescription for a three (3) month supply, sign the application, and mail it to TOBI Patient Support Program.

WHAT YOU HAVE TO DO: Stay in contact with your doctor's office. You will have to provide detailed financial information. You will have to sign the application.

WHERE THE MEDICATION GOES: The Cystic Fibrosis Pharmacy will mail one (1) box of medication to your home. The medication will not be sent to a P.O. Box.

AMOUNT GIVEN AT ONE TIME: A 28-day supply.

NO. OF REFILLS: 6

GENERAL INFORMATION: You can call between 9:00 am and 4:00 pm, Central Time, Monday through Friday.

MEDICATION AVAILABLE: TOBI

COMPANY: Pfizer Pharmaceuticals, Inc.

PROGRAM ADDRESS: Pfizer Prescription Assistance
P.O. Box 230970
Centerville, VA 20120

TOLL FREE PHONE NUMBER: 800-646-4455
ALTERNATIVE NUMBER: 800-438-1985, then #3, then #3

ELIGIBILITY: You cannot have insurance that provides prescription coverage and you must be ineligible for State Medicaid. Your income limit for a single member household is $12,000 ($1,000 per month) and for a family (undefined) $15,000 ($1,250 per month).

ENROLLMENT: Anyone can call for an enrollment application form.

FROM YOUR DOCTOR: Your doctor will have to write a letter on office stationery, stating your inability to pay for the medication, your medical need, attach a prescription, and mail it to Pfizer Prescription Assistance.

WHAT YOU HAVE TO DO: Stay in contact with your doctor's office. You will have to provide financial and insurance information.

WHERE THE MEDICATION GOES: The medication will be sent to your doctor's office. The medication will not be sent to a P.O. Box.

AMOUNT GIVEN AT ONE TIME: Usually a 90-day supply.

GENERAL INFORMATION: You can call between 8:30 am and 5:30 pm, Eastern Time, Monday through Friday.

MEDICATIONS AVAILABLE: Antivert, Antivert 25 mg Tabs, Antivert 50 mg Tabs, Atarax Tabs, Atarax Syrup, Cardura, Diabinese, Feldene, Glucotrol, Glucotrol XL, Marinol, Minipress, Minizide, Navane Capsules, Navane Concentrate, Norvasc, Oramorph SR, Procardia, Procardia XL, Renese, Roxanol, Roxanol 100, Sinequan Capsules, Sinequan Oral Concentrate, Tikosyn, Trovan, Viagra, Vibra-Tabs, Vibramycin, Viramune, Vistaril Tabs, Vistaril Capsules, Vistaril Oral Concentrate, Zoloft, Zyrtec Tabs, Zyrtec Syrup

COMPANY: Pfizer Pharmaceuticals

PROGRAM ADDRESS: Aricept Patient Assistance Program
                                        P.O. Box 25457
                                        Alexandria, VA 22313-5457

TOLL FREE PHONE NUMBER: 800-226-2072

ELIGIBILITY: You cannot have insurance that provides prescription coverage and you must be ineligible for State Medicaid. Your income for a single household must be less than $25,000 per year ($2,083 per month). If you have a dependent, you must earn less than $40,000 per year ($3,333 per month).

ENROLLMENT: Anyone can call for an enrollment application form. At the time of enrollment, they will need your income and insurance information. It is required. The enrollment application will only be sent to your physician.

FROM YOUR DOCTOR: Your doctor will complete the application, agrees you have no prescription coverage, signs the application, and mails (or faxes) it to Aricept Patient Assistance Program. A prescription is part of the enrollment application.

WHAT YOU HAVE TO DO: Stay in contact with your doctor's office. You have already provided financial and insurance information.

WHERE THE MEDICATION GOES: The medication will be sent to your doctor's office. The medication will not be sent to a P.O. Box.

AMOUNT GIVEN AT ONE TIME: Usually a 90-day supply.

GENERAL INFORMATION: You can call between 8:30 am and 5:30 pm, Eastern Time, Monday through Friday. Pfizer & Eisai, Inc., will include information on local and national Alzheimer's resources for caregivers and patients.

MEDICATION AVAILABLE: Aricept

COMPANY: Pfizer, Inc.

PROGRAM ADDRESS: Pfizer, Inc.
Patient Assistance Program
1101 King St.
Suite 600
Alexandria, VA 22314

TOLL FREE PHONE NUMBER: 800-869-9979

ELIGIBILITY: You cannot have insurance that provides prescription coverage, be involved in any other AIDS prescription programs and you must be ineligible for State Medicaid. Your income limit for a single household is less than $25,000 per year ($2,083 per month). If you have a dependent, you must earn less than $40,000 per year ($3,333 per month). You must be a legal resident of the U.S.A.

ENROLLMENT: Anyone can call for an enrollment application form. At the time of enrollment, Pfizer will require your name, date of birth, and the name and address of the treating physician. This application is patient-specific and will only be sent to the doctor office.

FROM YOUR DOCTOR: Your doctor will complete the application, attach a prescription (if necessary), sign the application, and mail it to Pfizer, Inc., Patient Assistance Program.

WHAT YOU HAVE TO DO: Stay in contact with your doctor's office. You will have to provide financial information.

WHERE THE MEDICATION GOES: The medication will be sent to your doctor's office. The medication will not be sent to a P.O. Box.

AMOUNT GIVEN AT ONE TIME: Usually a 90-day supply.

GENERAL INFORMATION: You can call between 8:30 am and 5:30 pm, Eastern Time, Monday through Friday. The Zithromax program is to assist patients taking 1200 mg weekly for the prevention of MAC. The medication must be for outpatient use.

MEDICATIONS AVAILABLE: Diflucan Oral Suspension, Diflucan Tabs, Zithromax Tabs, Zithromax Capsules, Zithromax Oral Suspension

COMPANY: Pharmacia & Upjohn

PROGRAM ADDRESS: RxMAP
                             P.O. Box 29043
                             Phoenix, AZ 8503

TOLL FREE PHONE NUMBER: 800-242-7014
                                    (For self-administered drugs)
                                    800-366-5570
                                    (For non-self-administered drugs)
FAX NUMBER: 602-314-7163

ELIGIBILITY: Call the appropriate the 800 Number (see pg. 212) to determine eligibility. You cannot have insurance that provides prescription coverage and you must be ineligible for State Medicaid. RxMAP is for patients with a **short-term** financial hardship with no other funding.

ENROLLMENT: Anyone can call for an enrollment application form.

FROM YOUR DOCTOR: Your doctor will complete Section 2 of the application, attach a prescription (if necessary), sign the application, and mail it to RxMAP.

WHAT YOU HAVE TO DO: Stay in contact with your doctor's office.

WHERE THE MEDICATION GOES: The following medication will be sent to your doctor's office: Adriamycin, Adrucil, Bleomycin, Camptosar, Cytosar-U, Depo-Provera, Fragmin Idamycin, Neosar, Toposar, Vincsar PFS, Zanosar, Zinecard. The medication will not be sent to a P.O. Box.

The following medication will be obtained through a pharmacy with a card you are provided with by RxMAP at the time of acceptance: Caverject, Dostinex, Emcyt, Estring, Halotestin, Cleocin, Mirapex, Mycobutin, Rescriptor, Xalatan. There is a $5.00 dispensing fee for these medications.

AMOUNT GIVEN AT ONE TIME: Pharmacy card is good for 6 months of 30-day increments. Fragmin is shipped in 14-day increments. Direct shipment: send in 30-days supply

GENERAL INFORMATION: They also have assistance available to help with reimbursement issues denials from insurance companies, coverage, billing, etc.

Oncology medicines: call 800-808-9111 between 8:30 am and 5:30 pm, Eastern Time, Monday through Friday

For Rescriptor: call 800-711-0807 between 9:00 am and 6:00 pm, Eastern Time, Monday through Friday.

For Genotropin: call 800-645-1280. It is a 24-hour line. Genotropin is available through Bridge Program during the period when the insurance claim is being resolved.

MEDICATIONS AVAILABLE: Adriamycin, Adrucil, Aromasin, Bleomycin, Camptosar, Caverject, Cytosar-U, Depo-Provera Injection, Depo-Provera Suppositories, Detrol, Dostinex, Ellence, Emcyt, Estring Capsules, Estring Vaginal Ring, Fragmin, Glyset, Halotestin, Idamycin, Mirapex, Mycobutin, Neosar, Pletal, Rescriptor, Toposar, Vincsar PFS, Xalatan, Zanosar, Zinecard

COMPANY: Proctor & Gamble Pharmaceuticals

PROGRAM ADDRESS: Proctor & Gamble Pharmaceuticals
Patient Assistance Program
17 Eaton Ave.
Norwich, NY 13815

TOLL FREE PHONE NUMBER: 800-830-9049

ELIGIBILITY: You cannot have insurance that provides prescription coverage and you must be ineligible for State Medicaid. Your income must fall below the Federal Poverty Guideline (see pg. 249-250). If your income is above the Federal Poverty Guideline, but your medical expense brings your income below the Federal Poverty Guideline; Proctor & Gamble will consider this.

ENROLLMENT: Anyone can call for an enrollment application form. You will be required to give financial and insurance information at the time of the call. Proctor & Gamble will decide if you qualify when you call. If you do qualify, the enrollment application will be mailed to your doctor.

FROM YOUR DOCTOR: Your doctor will complete the application, attach a prescription (if necessary), sign the application, and mail it to Proctor & Gamble.

WHAT YOU HAVE TO DO: Stay in contact with your doctor's office.

WHERE THE MEDICATION GOES: The medication can be sent directly to your home as long as someone is there to sign for the delivery. The medication will not be sent to a P.O. Box.

AMOUNT GIVEN AT ONE TIME: Usually a 90-day supply.

NO. OF REFILLS: You will send in a mailer for another 90-day supply. This should be done about four (4) weeks before running out of the medication.

GENERAL INFORMATION: You can call between 8:00 am and 5:00 pm, Eastern Time, Monday through Friday. This program has very strict guidelines.

MEDICATIONS AVAILABLE: Asacol, Dantrium, Didronel, Macrobid, Macrodantin

COMPANY: Purdue Frederick Company

PROGRAM ADDRESS: Purdue Frederick Company
                                     100 Connecticut Ave.
                                     Norwalk, CT 06850-3590

TOLL FREE PHONE NUMBER: 800-633-4741
ALTERNATIVE NUMBER: 203-853-0123
FAX NUMBER: 203-838-1576

ELIGIBILITY: You cannot have insurance that provides prescription coverage and you must be ineligible for State Medicaid.

ENROLLMENT: You doctor's office must call to start the process. The company representative will bring the application to the doctor's office.

FROM YOUR DOCTOR: Your doctor will complete the application, attach a prescription, signs the application, and notifies the company representative.

WHAT YOU HAVE TO DO: Stay in contact with your doctor's office. You will have to complete your part of the enrollment application. They will want financial and insurance information.

WHERE THE MEDICATION GOES: The medication will be sent to your doctor's office. The medication will not be sent to a P.O. Box.

AMOUNT GIVEN AT ONE TIME: Usually a 30-day supply.

GENERAL INFORMATION: You can call between 9:00 am and 4:00 pm, Eastern Time, Monday through Friday.

MEDICATIONS AVAILABLE: MS Contin, OxyContin

COMPANY: Rhone Poulenc Rorer, Inc.

PROGRAM ADDRESS: Rhone Poulenc Rorer, Inc.
                          Medical Affairs Indigent Access Program
                          Mail Stop P.O. 4C29
                          Box 5094
                          Collegeville, PA 19426-0998

TOLL FREE PHONE NUMBER: 800-340-7502

ELIGIBILITY: You cannot have insurance that provides prescription coverage and you must be ineligible for State Medicaid.

ENROLLMENT: Anyone can call for an enrollment application form.

FROM YOUR DOCTOR: Your doctor will complete the application, attach a prescription (if necessary), sign the application, and mail it to Rhone Poulenc Rorer, Inc.

WHAT YOU HAVE TO DO: Stay in contact with your doctor's office. You will have to provide financial and insurance information. You must sign the enrollment application.

WHERE THE MEDICATION GOES: The medication will be sent to your doctor's office. The medication will not be sent to a P.O. Box.

AMOUNT GIVEN AT ONE TIME: Usually a 90-day supply.

GENERAL INFORMATION: You will have to have a copy of rejection from Medicaid. This letter will have to accompany each new application (every 90 days). You can call between 9:00 am and 4:00 pm, Eastern Time, Monday through Friday.

MEDICATIONS AVAILABLE: Azmacort Inhaler Aerosol, Hygroton, Intal Inhaler, Intel Nebulizer Solution, Lovenox, Lozol, Nasacort AQ Inhaler, Nasacort AQ Nasal Spray, Nitrolingual Spray, Penetrex, Slo-Bid Gyrocaps, Slo-Phyllin GG Capsules, Slo-Phyllin GG Syrup, Slo-Phyllin Syrup, Slo-Phyllin Syrup 80, Slo-Phyllin Tablets, Tilade Inhaler, Tussar Syrup, Zagam

COMPANY: Rhone Poulenc Rorer, Inc.

PROGRAM ADDRESS: Rhone Poulenc Rorer, Inc.
                  Oncology Products
                  PACT Program
                  1101 King St.
                  Suite 600
                  Alexandria, VA 22314

TOLL FREE PHONE NUMBER: 800-996-6626

ELIGIBILITY: You cannot have insurance that provides prescription coverage and you must be ineligible for State Medicaid.

ENROLLMENT: You doctor will have to call for an enrollment application form. The doctor will provide the PACT Program with your name, address, telephone number, social security number, and date of birth. The enrollment application will be sent to your doctor.

FROM YOUR DOCTOR: Your doctor will complete the application, attach a prescription (if necessary), sign the application, and mail it to the PACT Program.

WHAT YOU HAVE TO DO: Stay in contact with your doctor's office.

WHERE THE MEDICATION GOES: The medication will be sent to your doctor's office. The medication will not be sent to a P.O. Box.

AMOUNT GIVEN AT ONE TIME: Depends on the type of therapy.

GENERAL INFORMATION: You will have to reapply after every four (4) treatments. You can call between 9:00 am and 4:00 pm, Eastern Time, Monday through Friday.

MEDICATIONS AVAILABLE: Gliadel Wafers, Oncaspar, Taxotere

COMPANY: Roberts Pharmaceutical

PROGRAM ADDRESS: Roberts Pharmaceutical
                       4 Industrial Way West
                       Eastontown, NJ 07724

ALTERNATIVE NUMBER: 800-828-2088

ELIGIBILITY: You cannot have insurance that provides prescription coverage and you must be ineligible for State Medicaid. There are income guidelines you must meet.

ENROLLMENT: Your doctor's office should call for an enrollment application form. The enrollment application will be faxed to your doctor.

FROM YOUR DOCTOR: Your doctor will complete the application, attach a prescription (if necessary), sign the application, and fax it to Roberts Pharmaceutical.

WHAT YOU HAVE TO DO: Stay in contact with your doctor's office. You may have to provide financial and insurance information.

WHERE THE MEDICATION GOES: The medication will be sent to your doctor's office. The medication will not be sent to a P.O. Box.

AMOUNT GIVEN AT ONE TIME: Usually a 90-day supply.

GENERAL INFORMATION: They do have programs for Agrylin for individuals not meeting the original income guidelines. You can call between 9:00 am and 4:00 pm, Eastern Time, Monday through Friday.

MEDICATIONS AVAILABLE: Agrylin, Pentasa, ProAmatine

COMPANY: Roche Labs

PROGRAM ADDRESS: Roche Labs
                             Medical Needs Program
                             340 Kingsland St.
                             Nutley, NJ 07110-1199

TOLL FREE PHONE NUMBER: 800-285-4484
FAX NUMBER: 703-518-4222

ELIGIBILITY: You cannot have insurance that provides prescription coverage and you must be ineligible for State Medicaid.

ENROLLMENT: Your doctor's office must call for an enrollment application form. At the time of the call, your doctor will need your financial and insurance information.

FROM YOUR DOCTOR: Your doctor will complete the enrollment application (your doctor's DEA number must be on the enrollment application), attach a prescription (if necessary), sign the application, and mail it to Roche Labs Medical Needs Program.

WHAT YOU HAVE TO DO: Stay in contact with your doctor's office. You will have to provide financial and insurance information.

WHERE THE MEDICATION GOES: The medication will be sent to your doctor's office. The medication will not be sent to a P.O. Box.

AMOUNT GIVEN AT ONE TIME: This varies according to what medication is involved—usually a 90-day supply.

GENERAL INFORMATION: You can call between 9:00 am and 4:00 pm, Eastern Time, Monday through Friday. Some of Roche's programs are quite simple to qualify for and some of the programs are quite difficult to qualify for.

Special phone numbers to use for specific medications:

CellCept:	800-772-5790
Cytovene:	800-282-7780, then #1
HIVID:	800-285-4484, then #2
Invirase:	800-282-7780
Roferon-A:	800-443-6676
Tamiflu:	800-285-4484
Tasmar:	800-285-4484
Xenline:	800-260-7785
Xeloda:	800-443-6676

MEDICATIONS AVAILABLE: Accuretic, Accutane, Anaprox DS Tabs, Anaprox Tabs, Bactrim DS Tabs, Bactrim Pediatric Suspension, Bactrim Tabs, Berocca, Berocca Plus, Bumex, Cardene, Cardene SR, CellCept Tabs, CellCept Capsules, CellCept Oral Suspension, Cytovene, Demadex, EC Naprosyn Tabs, Fluorouracil, Fortovase, FUDR, Gantanol, HIVID, Invirase, Klonopin, Kytril, Larodopa, Levodopa, Levo-Dromoran, Librax, Limbitrol, Limbitrol DS, Naprosyn, Naprosyn Capsules, Nasalide, Quarzan, Rocaltrol Tabs, Rocaltrol Capsules, Rocephin, Roferon-A, Soriatane, Tamiflu, Tasmar, Ticlid, Trimpex, Valium, Vesanoid, Xeloda, Xenline

COMPANY: Roxane Laboratories, Inc.

PROGRAM ADDRESS: Roxane Laboratories, Inc.
1101 King St.
Suite 600
Alexandria, VA 22314

TOLL FREE PHONE NUMBER: 800-274-8651
ALTERNATIVE NUMBER: 800-848-0120

ELIGIBILITY: You cannot have insurance that provides prescription coverage and you must be ineligible for State Medicaid.

ENROLLMENT: Anyone can call for an enrollment application form.

FROM YOUR DOCTOR: Your doctor will complete the enrollment application, attach a prescription (if necessary), sign the application, and mail it to Roxane Laboratories, Inc.

WHAT YOU HAVE TO DO: Stay in contact with your doctor's office. You will have to provide detailed financial information.

WHERE THE MEDICATION GOES: You will be sent a pharmacy card. You will take the card and a prescription to a participating pharmacy to have the prescription filled.

AMOUNT GIVEN AT ONE TIME: A 30-day supply. You will receive four (4) pharmacy cards, three (3) times during the year.

GENERAL INFORMATION: You can call between 9:00 am and 4:00 pm, Eastern Time, Monday through Friday. Marinol 2.5 mg capsules must be ordered in bottles of 60.

MEDICATIONS AVAILABLE: Marinol, Oramorph SR 30 mg, Oramorph SR 60 mg, Oramorph SR 100 mg, Roxanol 20 ml., Roxanol 120 ml, Roxanol 100 Oral Concentrate, Viramune Oral Suspension

COMPANY: Sankyo Pharmaceutical

PROGRAM ADDRESS: Sankyo Pharmaceutical
                        Open Care Program
                        P.O. Box 8409
                        Somerville, NJ 08876

TOLL FREE PHONE NUMBER: 866-268-7327

ELIGIBILITY: You cannot have insurance that provides prescription coverage and you must be ineligible for State Medicaid. You must be a legal U.S. resident. Household income guidelines: For a household of one (1) $15,462.00 per year ($1,288.00 per month), for a household of two (2): $20,898.00 per year ($1,741.00 per month), for a household of three (3) $26,334.00 per year ($2194.00 per month).

ENROLLMENT: Anyone can call for an enrollment application form.

FROM YOUR DOCTOR: Your doctor will complete the enrollment application, attach a prescription (if necessary), sign the application, and mail it to Sankyo Pharmaceutical.

WHAT YOU HAVE TO DO: Stay in contact with your doctor's office. You will have to provide detailed financial information. You **MUST CALL 886-268-7327** before mailing the application.

WHERE THE MEDICATION GOES: The medication will be sent to your doctor's office. The medication will not be sent to a P.O. Box.

AMOUNT GIVEN AT ONE TIME: The first shipment is a two (2) month supply. Then a three (3) month supply for a total of 11 months.

GENERAL INFORMATION: You can call between 9:00 am and 4:00 pm, Eastern Time, Monday through Friday.

MEDICATIONS AVAILABLE: WelChol

COMPANY: Sanofi Pharmaceuticals, Inc.

PROGRAM ADDRESS: Sanofi Pharmaceuticals, Inc.
                        Needy Patient Program
                        Product Information
                        Dept., 7th Floor
                        90 Park Ave.
                        New York, NY 10016

TOLL FREE PHONE NUMBER: 800-446-6267
ALTERNATIVE NUMBER: 212-551-4000
FAX NUMBER: 212-551-4902

ELIGIBILITY: You cannot have insurance that provides prescription coverage and you must be ineligible for State Medicaid. Your total household income for a single person must be below $10,300 per year ($858 per month), for a household of two (2) your income must be below $13,825 ($1,152 per month), they have guidelines up to households of 12. **You can only be on the program for six (6) months in any given year.**

ENROLLMENT: Your doctor's office should call for an enrollment application form.

FROM YOUR DOCTOR: Your doctor will complete the application, attach a prescription (if necessary), sign the application, and mail it to Sanofi Pharmaceuticals, Inc.

WHAT YOU HAVE TO DO: Stay in contact with your doctor's office.

WHERE THE MEDICATION GOES: The medication will be sent to your doctor's office. The medication will not be sent to a P.O. Box.

AMOUNT GIVEN AT ONE TIME: Usually a 90-day supply.

GENERAL INFORMATION: Each doctor can have only **six (6) patients** per year enrolled in the program. You can call between 9:00 am and 4:00 pm, Eastern Time, Monday through Friday.

MEDICATIONS AVAILABLE Aralen, Danocrine, Drisdol, Hytakerol, Mytelase, NegGram Caplets, NegGram Suspension, pHisoHex, Plaquenil, Primaquine, Skelid

COMPANY: Schein Pharmaceuticals

PROGRAM ADDRESS: Schein Pharmaceutical, Inc.
                     100 Campus Drive
                     Florham Park, NJ 07932

TOLL FREE PHONE NUMBER: 973-593-5500

ELIGIBILITY: You cannot have insurance that provides prescription coverage and you must be ineligible for State Medicaid. You must be a U.S. citizen with a gross household income of less than $25,000 per year ($2,083 per month).

ENROLLMENT: Your doctor's office should call for an enrollment application form.

FROM YOUR DOCTOR: Your doctor will complete the application, attach a prescription (if necessary), your current lab reports must be included, sign the application, and mail it to Schein Pharmaceuticals.

WHAT YOU HAVE TO DO: Stay in contact with your doctor's office.

WHERE THE MEDICATION GOES: The medication will be sent to your doctor's office. The medication will not be sent to a P.O. Box.

AMOUNT GIVEN AT ONE TIME: Usually a 90-day supply.

GENERAL INFORMATION: Once you are on the program, your doctor just sends current (within 30 days) lab reports to Schein Pharmaceuticals.

GENERAL INFORMATION: You can call between 9:00 am and 4:00 pm, Eastern Time, Monday through Friday.

MEDICATIONS AVAILABLE: Ferrlecit, Infed

COMPANY: Schering Corporation

PROGRAM ADDRESS: Schering Labs/Key Pharmaceuticals
                    Pt. Assistance Program
                    P.O. Box 52122
                    Phoenix, AZ 85072

TOLL FREE PHONE NUMBER: 800-656-9485
ALTERNATIVE NUMBER: 800-222-7579

ELIGIBILITY: You cannot have insurance that provides prescription coverage and you must be ineligible for State Medicaid. They have income guidelines but would not be specific only that your income must be under the Federal Poverty Guideline (see pg. 249-250).

ENROLLMENT: Your doctor's office should call for an enrollment application form.

FROM YOUR DOCTOR: Your doctor will complete the application, attach a prescription (if necessary), sign the application, and mail it to Schering Labs/Key Pharmaceuticals.

WHAT YOU HAVE TO DO: Stay in contact with your doctor's office. You will have to provide detailed financial and insurance information.

WHERE THE MEDICATION GOES: The medication will be sent to your doctor's office. The medication will not be sent to a P.O. Box.

AMOUNT GIVEN AT ONE TIME: Usually a 90-day supply.

GENERAL INFORMATION: You can call between 9:00 am and 4:00 pm, Mountain Time, Monday through Friday.

MEDICATIONS AVAILABLE: Celestone, Claritin D-12 Retabs, Claritin Retabs, Claritin Syrup, Claritin Tabs, Diprolene Cream, Diprolene Gel, Diprolene Lotion, Diprosone Cream, Diprosone Lotion, Diprosone Ointment, Elocon Cream, Elocon Gel, Elocon Lotion, Estinyl, Etrafon Forte Tabs, Eulexin, Fareston, Fulvicin, Garamycin Cream, Garamycin Gel, Garamycin Ophthalmic Solution, Imdur, InspirEase System, Intron-A, K-Dur, Lotrimin Cream, Lotrimin Lotion, Lotrimin Topical Ointment, Lotrisone Cream, Meticorten, Miradon, Naqua, Nasonex Nasal Spray, Nitro-Dur, Normodyne Tabs, Normodyne Injectable, Optimine, Permitil Oral Concentrate, Polaramine Expectorant, Polaramine Repetabs, Polaramine Syrup, Polaramine Tabs, Proventil (All Forms), Sebizon, Theo-Dur, Trilafon Tabs, Trilafon Concentrate, Uni-Dur, Vancenase AQ 0.04% Nasal Spray, Vancenase AQ 0.08% Nasal Spray, Vanceril Inhalation Aerosol

COMPANY: Schering-Plough Oncology

PROGRAM ADDRESS: Schering-Plough Oncology
                      Commitment to Care Program
                      1250 Bay Hill Dr.
                      San Bruno, CA 94066

TOLL FREE PHONE NUMBER: 800-521-7157
FAX NUMBER: 800-683-7855

ELIGIBILITY: You cannot have insurance that provides prescription coverage and you must be ineligible for State Medicaid.

ENROLLMENT: Anyone can call for an enrollment application form. A company representative will interview you on the telephone to assess your financial need.

FROM YOUR DOCTOR: A company representative will call your doctor, to let them know what is needed from your doctor.

WHAT YOU HAVE TO DO: Stay in contact with your doctor's office.

WHERE THE MEDICATION GOES: Upon acceptance into the program, you will be given an identification number to take to your pharmacy with a prescription from your doctor. The pharmacy will bill Commitment to Care Program and dispenses the drug.

AMOUNT GIVEN AT ONE TIME: This depends on the medication.

GENERAL INFORMATION: In instances of melanoma, your doctor can call and the Schering-Plough Oncology will get you into the system as quickly as possible. Usually there is some co-pay amount unless you are totally indigent.

GENERAL INFORMATION: You can call between 9:00 am and 4:00 pm, Pacific Time, Monday through Friday.

MEDICATIONS AVAILABLE: Eulexin, Intron-A, Rebetron, Temodar

COMPANY: Scios, Inc.

PROGRAM ADDRESS: Scios, Inc.
                        820 West Maude Ave.
                        Sunnyvale, CA 94085

TOLL FREE PHONE NUMBER: 800-972-4670

ELIGIBILITY: You cannot have insurance that provides prescription coverage and you must be ineligible for State Medicaid.

ENROLLMENT: Your doctor needs to call the toll-free number between 8:00 am-5:00 pm, Pacific Time. This automated system will ask for the doctor's name and fax number. The enrollment application will be faxed to your doctor.

FROM YOUR DOCTOR: Your doctor will complete the application, attach a prescription for a 90-day supply, sign the application, and mail it to the address on the enrollment application.

WHAT YOU HAVE TO DO: Stay in contact with your doctor's office. You will be required to sign the form.

WHERE THE MEDICATION GOES: The medication will be sent to your doctor's office. The medication will not be sent to a P.O. Box.

AMOUNT GIVEN AT ONE TIME: Usually a 90-day supply.

MEDICATIONS AVAILABLE: Eskalith CR, Parnate, Stelazine, Thorazine

COMPANY: Searle & Company

PROGRAM ADDRESS: Searle & Company
                             Patients in Need Foundation
                             5200 Old Orchard Rd.
                             Skokie, IL 60077

TOLL FREE PHONE NUMBER: 800-542-2526
ALTERNATIVE NUMBER: 800-323-1603
FAX NUMBER: 708-470-6633

ELIGIBILITY: You cannot have insurance that provides prescription coverage and you must be ineligible for State Medicaid.

ENROLLMENT: Only your doctor's office can call for an enrollment application form.

FROM YOUR DOCTOR: Your doctor will complete the application, attach a prescription for a 30-day supply of a Searle brand name medication (this prohibits substitution), sign the application, and mail it to Searle & Co.

WHAT YOU HAVE TO DO: Stay in contact with your doctor's office.

WHERE THE MEDICATION GOES: Searle will send certificates or vouchers to doctor's office. Your doctor will give you the certificates or vouchers to take to your pharmacy. The pharmacy will provide the medication free.

AMOUNT GIVEN AT ONE TIME: Usually a 30-day supply.

GENERAL INFORMATION: Your doctor must call to register with the program. They must have your doctor's DEA number on file. You can call between 9:00 am and 4:00 pm, Central Time, Monday through Friday.

MEDICATIONS AVAILABLE: Aldactazide, Aldactone, Arthrotec, Calan, Calan SR, Celebrex 100 mg, Celebrex 200 mg, Covera-HS, Cytotec, Kerlone, Norpace, Norpace CR

COMPANY: Serono Laboratories

PROGRAM ADDRESS: Serono Laboratories
         Helping Hand Program
         100 Longwater Circle
         Norwell, ME 02061

TOLL FREE PHONE NUMBER: 800-283-8088
ALTERNATIVE NUMBER: 617-982-9000
FAX NUMBER: 617-982-1369

ELIGIBILITY: You cannot have insurance that provides prescription coverage and you must be ineligible for State Medicaid.

ENROLLMENT: Your doctor's office must call for an enrollment application form. The enrollment application will be sent to your doctor's office.

FROM YOUR DOCTOR: Your doctor will complete the application, attach a prescription (if necessary), sign the application, and mail it to Serono Laboratories.

WHAT YOU HAVE TO DO: Stay in contact with your doctor's office.

WHERE THE MEDICATION GOES: The medication will be sent to your doctor's office. The medication will not be sent to a P.O. Box.

AMOUNT GIVEN AT ONE TIME: Usually a 90-day supply.

GENERAL INFORMATION: You can call between 9:00 am and 4:00 pm, Eastern Time, Monday through Friday.

MEDICATIONS AVAILABLE: Metrodin, Urofollitropin

COMPANY: Shire Pharmaceuticals

PROGRAM ADDRESS: Shire Pharmaceuticals
                   Patient Assistance Program
                   P.O. Box 698
                   Somerville NJ 08876

ALTERNATIVE NUMBER: 908-203-0657

ELIGIBILITY: You cannot have insurance that provides prescription coverage and you must be ineligible for State Medicaid. There are income guidelines depending on the drug.

ENROLLMENT: Anyone can call for an enrollment application form. They will need the doctor's name and address. Shire Pharmaceuticals will send the enrollment application to your doctor's office.

FROM YOUR DOCTOR: Your doctor will complete the application, attach a prescription (if necessary), sign the application, and mail it to Shire Pharmaceuticals.

WHAT YOU HAVE TO DO: Stay in contact with your doctor's office.

WHERE THE MEDICATION GOES: The medication will be sent to your doctor's office. The medication will not be sent to a P.O. Box.

AMOUNT GIVEN AT ONE TIME: Usually a 90-day supply.

GENERAL INFORMATION: If you only have Medicare, Shire Pharmaceuticals will need you to provide a copy of your Medicare card and a written statement saying you have no prescription coverage. Shire Pharmaceuticals also has a cost-share program for individuals who don't meet the eligibility guidelines for assistance. You can call between 9:00 am and 4:00 pm, Eastern Time, Monday through Friday.

MEDICATIONS AVAILABLE: Agrylin, Ethmozine, Fareston, Pentasa, ProAmatine

COMPANY: SmithKline Beecham, Inc.

PROGRAM ADDRESS: SmithKline Beecham, Inc.
                         Access to Care Program
                         P.O. Box 2564
                         Maryland Heights, MO 63043

TOLL FREE PHONE NUMBER: 800-546-0420 (for forms)
ALTERNATIVE NUMBER: 800-729-4544 (for information)

ELIGIBILITY: You cannot have insurance that provides prescription coverage and you must be ineligible for State Medicaid. You must be a U.S. resident with an annual household income of less than $25,000 per year ($2,083 per month).

ENROLLMENT: Your doctor's office must call for an enrollment application form. This is a carbonless form (it cannot be copied) and will be mailed to your doctor.

FROM YOUR DOCTOR: Your doctor will complete the application, attach a prescription (if necessary), sign the application, and mail it to SmithKline Beecham, Inc.

WHAT YOU HAVE TO DO: Stay in contact with your doctor's office. You will have to provide financial and insurance information.

WHERE THE MEDICATION GOES: The medication will be sent directly to you. The medication will not be sent to a P.O. Box.

AMOUNT GIVEN AT ONE TIME: Usually a 90-day supply.

NO. OF REFILLS: After 90 days, your doctor needs to send a new application form.

GENERAL INFORMATION: Products must be for an FDA-indicated use, **NO OFF LABEL USAGE.** The enrollment packet consists of 20 forms. You can call between 9:00 am and 4:00 pm, Central Time, Monday through Friday.

MEDICATIONS AVAILABLE: Amoxil Chewable Tabs, Amoxil Concentrate, Amoxil Tabs, Augmentin Chewable Tabs, Augmentin Oral Concentrate, Avandia, Bactroban Cream, Bactroban Nasal, Compazine Tabs, Compazine Spansules, Compazine Suppositories, Compazine Syrup, Coreg, Dyazide, Famvir, Ornade, Paxil, Relafen, Ridaura, Stelazine Tabs, Stelazine Concentrate, Tagamet Tabs, Tagamet Liquid

COMPANY: Solvay Pharmaceuticals, Inc.

PROGRAM ADDRESS: Solvay Patient Assistance Program
                           c/o Phoenix Marketing Group
                           One Phoenix Drive
                           Lincoln Park, NJ 07035

TOLL FREE PHONE NUMBER: 800-788-9277
ALTERNATIVE NUMBER: 770-578-9000

ELIGIBILITY: You cannot have insurance that provides prescription coverage and you must be ineligible for State Medicaid. You must be a U.S. resident.

ENROLLMENT: Your doctor's office should call for an enrollment application. Solvay Pharmaceuticals will send the enrollment application to your doctor's office.

FROM YOUR DOCTOR: Your doctor will complete the application, attach a prescription (if necessary), sign the application, and mail it to Solvay Pharmaceutical, Inc.

WHAT YOU HAVE TO DO: Stay in contact with your doctor's office. You will have to provide detailed financial and insurance information.

WHERE THE MEDICATION GOES: The medication will be sent to your doctor's office. The medication will not be sent to a P.O. Box.

AMOUNT GIVEN AT ONE TIME: Usually a 90-day supply.

GENERAL INFORMATION: You can call between 9:00 am and 4:00 pm, Eastern Time, Monday through Friday.

MEDICATIONS AVAILABLE: Creon, Estratab, Estratest, Estratest HS, Lithobid, Luvox 25 mg Tabs, Luvox 50 mg Tabs, Luvox 100 mg Tabs, Rowasa Enema, Treveten

COMPANY: Takeda Pharmaceuticals, America

PROGRAM ADDRESS: Express Scripts
Specialty Distribution Services
Attn: Takeda PAP Program
P.O. Box 66552
St. Louis, MO 63166

TOLL FREE PHONE NUMBER: 877-825-3327
ALTERNATIVE NUMBER: 877-582-5332
FAX NUMBER: 800-497-0928

ELIGIBILITY: You cannot have insurance that provides prescription coverage and you must be ineligible for State Medicaid. Your income must be under 200% of Federal Poverty Guideline (see pg. 249-250). You must be a legal U.S. Citizen.

ENROLLMENT: Your doctor's office should call for the enrollment application. It will be faxed to your doctor's office.

FROM YOUR DOCTOR: Your doctor will complete the application, attach a prescription for a 90-day supply, sign the application, and fax it to Express Scripts.

WHAT YOU HAVE TO DO: Stay in contact with your doctor's office. You will have to provide financial and insurance information. You must sign the enrollment application.

WHERE THE MEDICATION GOES: The medication will be sent to your doctor's office. The medication will not be sent to a P.O. Box.

AMOUNT GIVEN AT ONE TIME: Usually a 90-day supply.

GENERAL INFORMATION: You can call between 9:00 am and 4:00 pm, Central Time, Monday through Friday.

MEDICATION AVAILABLE: Actos

COMPANY: TAP Pharmaceuticals

PROGRAM ADDRESS: TAP Pharmaceuticals
                        Compassionate Program
                        2355 Waukegan Rd.
                        Deerfield, Ill 60015

TOLL FREE PHONE NUMBER: 800-453-8438
ALTERNATIVE NUMBER: 800-621-1020
FAX NUMBER: 847-267-5657

ELIGIBILITY: You cannot have insurance that provides prescription coverage and you must be ineligible for State Medicaid.

ENROLLMENT: Your doctor's office should call for the enrollment application form. They will have to provide patient's name, diagnosis, doctor's name, doctor's DEA number, name of contact person, phone and a fax number.

FROM YOUR DOCTOR: Your doctor will complete the application, attach a prescription (if necessary), sign the application, and mail it to TAP Pharmaceuticals.

WHAT YOU HAVE TO DO: Stay in contact with your doctor's office. You will have to provide detailed financial and insurance information.

WHERE THE MEDICATION GOES: The medication will be sent to your doctor's office. The medication will not be sent to a P.O. Box.

AMOUNT GIVEN AT ONE TIME: This depends on each person's situation, the diagnosis and amount of Lupron you have already had.

GENERAL INFORMATION: You can call between 7:30 am and 5:00 pm, Central Time, Monday through Friday,

For the Prevacid Program: Call 800-830-1015

MEDICATIONS AVAILABLE: Lupron, Prevacid

COMPANY: UCB Pharmaceuticals, Inc.

PROGRAM ADDRESS: Medical Affairs Department
                              1950 Lake Park Drive
                              Smyrna GA 30080

TOLL FREE PHONE NUMBER: 800-477-7877 (then chose option 7)

ELIGIBILITY: You cannot have insurance that provides prescription coverage and you must be ineligible for State Medicaid. You must be a U.S. resident. Your household income for a single person must be less than $15,000 per year ($1,250 per month). If you have dependents, your household income must be less than $25,000 per year ($2,083 per month).

ENROLLMENT: Your doctor's office must call for an enrollment application form. UCB Pharmaceuticals, Inc., will send a package containing information including the enrollment application and re-enrollment application.

FROM YOUR DOCTOR: Your doctor will complete the application, attach a prescription (if necessary), sign the application, and mail it to UCB Pharmaceuticals, Inc. Your doctor must attach a letter on office stationery certifying the medication will be used for indicated use and dosage that conforms to product labeling. **Your doctor must include a diagnostic code.**

WHAT YOU HAVE TO DO: Stay in contact with your doctor's office. You will have to provide financial and insurance information. You must sign the enrollment application.

WHERE THE MEDICATION GOES: The medication will be sent to your doctor's office. The medication will not be sent to a P.O. Box.

AMOUNT GIVEN AT ONE TIME: Usually a 90-day supply.

GENERAL INFORMATION: You can call between 9:00 am and 4:00 pm, Eastern Time, Monday through Friday.

MEDICATION AVAILABLE: Keppra

COMPANY: Unimed Pharmaceuticals

PROGRAM ADDRESS: Anadrol-50
                            Patient Assistance Program
                            P.O. Box 222197
                            Charlotte, NC 28222-2197

TOLL FREE PHONE NUMBER: 800-256-8918
ALTERNATIVE NUMBER: 847-541-2525
FAX NUMBER: 800-276-9901

ELIGIBILITY: You cannot have insurance that provides prescription coverage and you must be ineligible for State Medicaid.

ENROLLMENT: Your doctor should call for an enrollment application form.

FROM YOUR DOCTOR: Your doctor will complete the application, attach a prescription (if necessary), sign the application, and fax it to Unimed Pharmaceuticals.

WHAT YOU HAVE TO DO: Stay in contact with your doctor's office. You will have to provide insurance and income information. Proof of income may be requested. You must sign the enrollment application.

WHERE THE MEDICATION GOES: The medication will be sent to your doctor's office. The medication will not be sent to a P.O. Box.

AMOUNT GIVEN AT ONE TIME: Usually a 90-day supply.

GENERAL INFORMATION: Call between 7:00 am and 6:00 pm, Eastern Time, Monday through Friday. The doctor can apply for the product on a one-time basis for new patient trial use.

MEDICATIONS AVAILABLE: Anadrol-50

COMPANY: Upsher-Smith

PROGRAM ADDRESS: Upsher-Smith
14905 23rd Ave. North
Minneapolis, MN 55447

TOLL FREE PHONE NUMBER: 800-654-2299

ELIGIBILITY: You cannot have insurance that provides prescription coverage and you must be ineligible for State Medicaid.

ENROLLMENT: Upsher-Smith does not have a formal program.

FROM YOUR DOCTOR: Your doctor will have to contact their sales representative in the area. Your doctor will write a letter on office stationery stating your need for the medication and your inability to purchase the medication.

WHAT YOU HAVE TO DO: Stay in contact with your doctor's office.

WHERE THE MEDICATION GOES: The medication will be sent to your doctor's office. The medication will not be sent to a P.O. Box.

AMOUNT GIVEN AT ONE TIME: Usually a 90-day supply.

MEDICATIONS AVAILABLE: AmLatin 12% Moisturizing Crème, AmLatin 12% Moisturizing Lotion, Klor-Con, Niacon, OMS Concentrate, Pacerome, Prevalite, RMS Suppositories, Slo-Niacin, SSKI Solution

COMPANY: U.S. Bioscience, Inc.

PROGRAM ADDRESS: U.S. Bioscience, Inc.
                         Reimbursement Program
                         c/o CRC
                         8990 Springbrook Drive,
                         Suite 200
                         Minneapolis, MN 55433

TOLL FREE PHONE NUMBER: 800-872-4672
ALTERNATIVE NUMBER: 612-832-0570
FAX NUMBER: 612-785-2709

ELIGIBILITY: You cannot have insurance that provides prescription coverage and you must be ineligible for State Medicaid.

ENROLLMENT: **For Hexalen:** Anyone can call for an enrollment application form. The enrollment application is sent to your doctor. It may be copied.

For Neutrexin: Anyone can call for an enrollment application form. The enrollment application is sent to your doctor. This form **may not** be copied; it is patient-specific.

FROM YOUR DOCTOR: Your doctor will complete the application, attach a prescription (if necessary), sign the application, and mail it to U.S. Bioscience, Inc.

WHAT YOU HAVE TO DO: Stay in contact with your doctor's office. You will have to provide detailed insurance and financial information. You must sign the form for Neutrexin but not for Hexalen.

WHERE THE MEDICATION GOES: The medication will be sent to your doctor's office. The medication will not be sent to a P.O. Box.

AMOUNT GIVEN AT ONE TIME: Hexalen: two (2) bottles of 100 pills (enough for one (1) course of therapy). Neutrexin: one (1) cycle of therapy per shipment

GENERAL INFORMATION: You can call between 9:00 am and 4:00 pm, Central Time, Monday through Friday.

MEDICATIONS AVAILABLE: Hexalen, Neutrexin

COMPANY: Westwood-Squibb Pharmaceuticals

PROGRAM ADDRESS: Westwood-Squibb Pharmaceuticals
                          Consumer Affairs Department
                          100 Forest Ave.
                          Buffalo NY 14213

TOLL FREE PHONE NUMBER: 800-333-0950

ELIGIBILITY: You cannot have insurance that provides prescription coverage and you must be ineligible for State Medicaid.

ENROLLMENT: There is no formal enrollment application form. Your doctor's office should call and explain your circumstances.

FROM YOUR DOCTOR Your doctor will write a letter on office letterhead stationery, explaining your financial and insurance situation. Your doctor should include a diagnosis, attach a prescription for a 90-day supply, and mail it to Westwood-Squibb Pharmaceuticals.

WHAT YOU HAVE TO DO: Stay in contact with your doctor's office.

WHERE THE MEDICATION GOES: The medication will be sent to your doctor's office. The medication will not be sent to a P.O. Box.

AMOUNT GIVEN AT ONE TIME: Usually a 90-day supply.

GENERAL INFORMATION: You can call between 9:00 am and 4:00 pm, Eastern Time, Monday through Friday.

MEDICATIONS AVAILABLE: Capitrol Shampoo, Eurax Lotion, Exelderm Cream, Exelderm Solution, Halog Cream, Halog Ointment, Halog Solution, Lac-Hydrin, T-Stat Topical Solution, Westcort Cream, Westcort Ointment

COMPANY: Westwood-Squibb Pharmaceuticals

PROGRAM ADDRESS: Westwood-Squibb Pharmaceuticals
                           Dovonex Patient Assistant Program
                           P.O. Box 1610
                           Alexandria, VA 22313

TOLL FREE PHONE NUMBER: 800-736-0003

ELIGIBILITY: You cannot have insurance that provides prescription coverage and you must be ineligible for State Medicaid.

ENROLLMENT: Your doctor's office will have to call for an enrollment application form. Westwood-Squibb will require at the time of registration your doctor's: tax ID number, social security number, DEA number, specialty, and office contact. Westwood-Squibb will also require: your name, social security number, address, telephone number, date of birth, number of people in your household, insurance information, financial information, and disability status.

FROM YOUR DOCTOR: Your doctor will complete the application, attach a prescription (if necessary), sign the application, and mail it to Westwood-Squibb Pharmaceuticals.

WHAT YOU HAVE TO DO: Stay in contact with your doctor's office. You will have to complete and sign the application.

WHERE THE MEDICATION GOES: The medication will be sent to your doctor's office. The medication will not be sent to a P.O. Box.

AMOUNT GIVEN AT ONE TIME: Usually a 90-day supply.

GENERAL INFORMATION: You can call between 9:00 am and 8:00 pm, Eastern Time, Monday through Friday.

MEDICATIONS AVAILABLE: Dovonex Cream, Dovonex Lotion, Dovonex Scalp Solution

COMPANY: Wyeth-Ayerst Laboratories

PROGRAM ADDRESS: Wyeth-Ayerst Laboratories
                            Professional Services IPP
                            P.O. Box 13806
                            Philadelphia, PA 19101

TOLL FREE PHONE NUMBER: 800-395-9938
ALTERNATIVE NUMBER: 800-568-9938

ELIGIBILITY: You cannot have insurance that provides prescription coverage and you must be ineligible for State Medicaid.

ENROLLMENT: Anyone can call for an enrollment application form.

FROM YOUR DOCTOR: Your doctor will complete the application, attach a prescription (if necessary), sign the application, and mail it to Wyeth-Ayerst Laboratories.

WHAT YOU HAVE TO DO: Stay in contact with your doctor's office. You must sign the enrollment application.

WHERE THE MEDICATION GOES: The medication will be sent to your doctor's office. The medication will not be sent to a P.O. Box.

AMOUNT GIVEN AT ONE TIME: Usually a 90-day supply.

GENERAL INFORMATION: Ativan and Serax are not covered. You can call between 9:00 am and 4:00 pm, Eastern Time, Monday through Friday.

MEDICATIONS AVAILABLE: Acebutolol HCL, Albuterol Sulfate, Antabuse, Artane, Atromid S, Auralgan Optic Solution, Aygestin, Cefaclor, Cimetidine, Clonidine HCL, Cordarone, Cycrin, Declomycin, Diamox Sequals, Diamox Tabs, Dicloxacillin, Digoxin in Tubex, Diltiazem HCL, Dimenhydrinate in Tubex, Dimetane, Diucardin, Donnatal, Effexor Tabs, Effexor XR, Entolase HP, Entozyme, Estradurin, Fenoprofen, Grisactin Tabs, Grisactin Capsules, Inderal, Inderal LA, Inderide, Inderide LA, ISMO, Isordil Sublingual Tabs, Isordil Tembids, Isordil Titradose, Lodine Tabs, Lodine Capsules, Lodine XL Tabs, Lodine XL Capsules, Methazolamide, Methotrexate, Methyldopa, Minocin, Mitrolan, Naproxen, Neptazane, Nistatin Suspension, Orudis, Oruvail, Pabalate, Phenergan (All Types), Phospholine Iodide, Prazosin Capsules, Prazosin HCL, Premarin, Premphase, Prempro, Promethazine HCL Syrup, Pronemia, Propylthiouracil, Pyrazinamide, Quinidex Extentabs, Quinidine Sulfate, Reglan, Rheumatrex, Robaxin, Robaxisal, Robicillin BK, Robimycin, Sectral, Selegiline, Sparine, Sulindac, Suprax, Surmontil, Tenex, Tetracycline, Thiosulfil Forte Tabs, Trecator-SC 250, Trihemic, Wyamycin S, Wytersin 4 mg, Zebeta, Ziac

Medication: _____

Phone Number: _____

Date I called: _____

Who I talked to: _____

Notes: _____

_____

_____

_____

_____

_____

_____

Medication: _____

Phone Number: _____

Date I called: _____

Who I talked to: _____

Notes: _____

_____

_____

_____

_____

_____

_____

Medication: _____

Phone Number: _____

Date I called: _____

Who I talked to: _____

Notes: _____

_____

_____

_____

_____

_____

_____

Medication: _____

Phone Number: _____

Date I called: _____

Who I talked to: _____

Notes: _____

_____

_____

_____

_____

_____

_____

Medication: _____

Phone Number: _____

Date I called: _____

Who I talked to: _____

Notes: _____

_____

_____

_____

_____

_____

_____

Medication: _____

Phone Number: _____

Date I called: _____

Who I talked to: _____

Notes: _____

_____

_____

_____

_____

_____

_____

Medication: _____

Phone Number: _____

Date I called: _____

Who I talked to: _____

Notes: _____

_____

_____

_____

_____

_____

_____

Medication: _____

Phone Number: _____

Date I called: _____

Who I talked to: _____

Notes: _____

_____

_____

_____

_____

_____

_____

Medication: _____

Phone Number: _____

Date I called: _____

Who I talked to: _____

Notes: _____

_____

_____

_____

_____

_____

_____

Medication: _____

Phone Number: _____

Date I called: _____

Who I talked to: _____

Notes: _____

_____

_____

_____

_____

_____

_____

Medication: _____

Phone Number: _____

Date I called: _____

Who I talked to: _____

Notes: _____

_____

_____

_____

_____

_____

_____

Medication: _____

Phone Number: _____

Date I called: _____

Who I talked to: _____

Notes: _____

_____

_____

_____

_____

_____

_____

Books Available From Robert D. Reed Publishers

Please include payment with orders. Send indicated book/s to:

Name:_____

Address:_____

City:_____ State:_____ Zip:_____

Phone:(____)_____ E-mail:_____

Titles and Authors	Unit Price
Free or Almost Free Prescription Medications by David Johnson	$19.95
House Calls: How we can all heal the world one visit at a time by Patch Adams, M.D.	11.95
LifeForce: A Dynamic Plan for Health, Vitality, and Weight Loss by Dr. Jeffrey S. McCombs, DC	11.95
Gotta Minute? The ABC's of Successful Living by Tom Massey, Ph.D., N.D.	9.95
Gotta Minute? Practical Tips for Abundant Living: The ABC's of Total Health by Tom Massey, Ph.D., N.D.	9.95
Gotta Minute? How to Look & Feel Great! by Marcia F. Kamph, M.S., D.C.	11.95
Gotta Minute? Yoga for Health, Relaxation & Well-being by Nirvair Singh Khalsa	9.95
A Kid's Herb Book For Children Of All Ages by Lesley Tierra, Acupuncturist and Herbalist	19.95
500 Tips For Coping With Chronic Illness by Pamela D. Jacobs, M.A.	11.95

Enclose a copy of this order form with payment for books. Send to the address below. Shipping & handling: $2.50 for first book plus $1.00 for each additional book. California residents add 8.5% sales tax. We offer discounts for large orders.

Please make checks payable to: Robert D. Reed Publishers. Total enclosed: $_____. See our website for more books!

Robert D. Reed Publishers
750 La Playa, Suite 647, San Francisco, CA 94121
Phone: 650-994-6570 • Fax: 650-994-6579
Email: 4bobreed@msn.com • www.rdrpublishers.com